Don't Eat the Oil!
The Health Consequences of Consuming "Vegetable" Oils

Thomas L. Copmann, MS., Ph.D.

The author of this book is not a physician and the ideas, procedures, and suggestions in this book are not intended as a substitute for the medical advice of a trained health professional. All matters regarding your health require medical supervision. Consult your physician before adopting the suggestions in this book, as well as about any condition that may require diagnosis or medical attention. The author and publisher disclaim any liability arising directly or indirectly from the use of this book.

DEDICATION

To my wife Kathleen, who's love and belief in me makes all things possible.
To my father Lyle D. Copmann who instilled within me my love of the written word.

Contents

Introduction

This book is a compilation of two and a half years of research based entirely on peer-reviewed publications. While I wasn't planning on publishing a book, the further I looked into the interrelationship of a number of major diseases, there slowly appeared to be a common denominator – the levels of polyunsaturated oils in our fatty tissues from consuming vegetable oils. Finally, the weight of evidence compelled me to write this book.

Polyunsaturated oils are a fairly new addition to the modern diet. Prior to their introduction at the turn of the century, cooking fats were mostly beef tallow and butter. Corn oil was introduced in 1911, followed by cottonseed, soybean, and rapeseed (Canola) oil labeled as "vegetable" oils. The fact is however, these oils have nothing in common with vegetables, but are the product of solvent extraction of oils from seeds.

The problem with these oils is their molecular structure. They are rich in polyunsaturated fats which means they have multiple double bonds between carbon atoms. Oxygen reacts with the double bonds in a process called *lipid peroxidation*. The end result is the formation of highly reactive free radicals which interact with cellular membranes, nuclear DNA, and deplete cells of their antioxidant defenses.

As you read the following chapters, the important thing to remember is exposing polyunsaturated fats to oxygen leads to free radical formation, while saturated fat cannot undergo this reaction because of their lack of double bonds. During the process of oil extraction, the oil is subject to high temperatures which accelerate the peroxidation reaction.

Polyunsaturated fats break down as their double bonds are exposed to oxygen. And heating accelerated this process. Therefore, lipid peroxidation is the degradation process involving the double bond(s) found in polyunsaturated fatty acids, causing a deterioration of food quality (odor, flavor, color, texture, toxicity). This is collectively known as turning "rancid". According to one analysis, a total of 130 volatile compounds were isolated from a piece of fried chicken alone!

As you digest the content of this book, I would ask you to keep an open mind, and then make your own decisions based on the totality of information. I ask this because a good deal of what you will be presented will be contrary with what you have read from *informed sources*. The web is full of simplified statement such as saturated fats are "bad" fats, or polyunsaturated fats are "good" fats. We will explore the origins of these statements, and show how our understandings have evolved. Unfortunately, older conclusions have a way of taking on a life of their own, and it is difficult to change what has become a culture brought on by successful marketing.

In summary, polyunsaturated fats are highly unstable and are readily oxidized to form toxic compounds that are implicated in most of our modern diseases (cardiovascular disease, cancer, obesity, immunological disorders, neurological disease processes, dysbiosis, lipofuscin, and premature aging). We will explore each of these in detail looking at mechanistic as well as epidemiological evidence.

1. The Elegant Complexity of Fats

To understand the impact of polyunsaturated fats on the function of cellular structures, we must first look at the structure and functions of fats. The term fat is used frequently both in every day conversation as well in scientific publications. In both cases, the term encompasses a large class of molecules with differing structures and functions. Unfortunately, results of numerous trials frequently do not take into account the complexity of the individual fat molecule, the three-dimensional structure, nor the degree conversion the molecule has undergone.

Fats serve four distinct functions: 1) the first and

most obvious is to serve as a means of storing energy; 2) they serve as the basic building blocks to cellular mem-

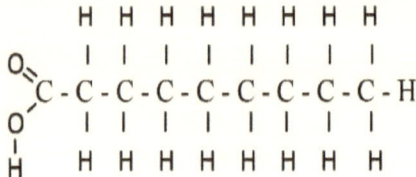

Figure 1: Fatty acid molecule

branes and structures; 3) certain fats serve as molecular messengers signaling systemic physiological changes (eicosanoids and hormones); and 4) to serve to insulate the body against thermal injury.

To review your high school chemistry, fats (or lipids) are compounds that are composed of carbon, hydrogen and oxygen molecules. The carbon atom is tetravalent, meaning it is capable of making four electrons available to form covalent chemical bonds with four adjacent atoms. The fatty acids are long, unbranched molecules containing 10 to 22 carbon atoms with the general formula seen in Figure 1.

The fatty acids have two ends, the carboxylic acid (-COOH) end, which is considered the head of the chain, or *alpha*, and the methyl (CH_3) end which is considered the tail of the chain, or *omega*. The way in which a fatty acid is named is determined by the location of the first double bond, counted from the methyl end (that is, the omega (ω-) or the n- end).

The head of the lipid molecule is a carboxylic acid group. Therefore, lipids are considered to be weak acids. Free fatty acids are rare in the cell due to their relative toxicity to cells. Fatty acids are typically found as components of larger lipid molecules. Free fatty acids are transported through the blood bound to serum albumin.

Saturated v Unsaturated Fats

Saturated fatty acids are lipid molecules whose carbon atoms are saturated with hydrogen. Most saturated fatty acids are straight hydrocarbon chains with an even number of carbon atoms. The most common fatty acids contain 12–22 carbon atoms. Saturated fats are commonly found in animals, and are solid at room temperature. Lard, suet, and butter are common saturated animal fats; coconut and palm oil are two saturated vegetable oils. Saturated fats are generally more stable than the unsaturated fats due to the lack of the double bond.

Monounsaturated and Polyunsaturated Fatty Acids

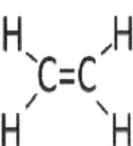

Figure 2: Monounsaturated fatty acid as characterized by the single double bond between the two carbon molecules.

Monounsaturated fatty acids have one carbon–carbon double bond. Oleic acid, present in olive oil, is a monounsaturated fat. When more than one area of the carbon chain contain double bonds, the fat is said to be polyunsaturated. Linoleic acid, an essential fatty

3

acid found in safflower oil, soybean oil, and other vegetable oils, is an example of a polyunsaturated fat. Other
oils of this category include peanut, corn, and cottonseed oils.

This difference in
double bonds is ex-
tremely important in un-
derstanding the differ-
ences in saturated and unsaturated fats and their effect on human metabo-
lism. Unsaturated fats are
unstable at room temper-
ature and sensitive to interaction with oxygen,
light, and heat. With the
increase of unsaturation, there is increase in primary oxidation products. These oxidation products incorporate
into various aspects of the cell and can be extremely
toxic, as we will see in chapter 3.

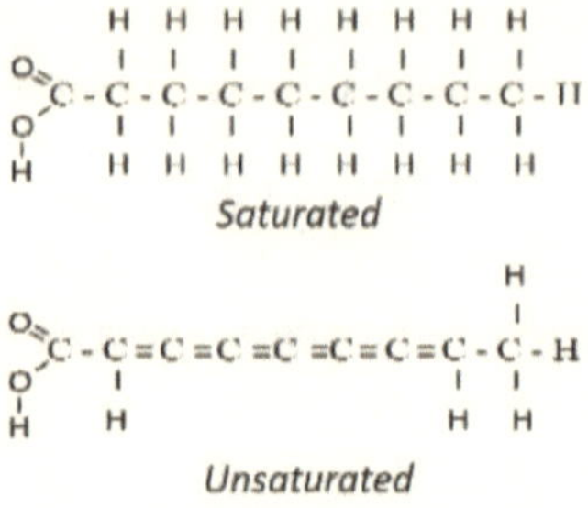

*Figure 3: Saturated fatty acid vs.
Polyunsaturated fatty acid. Polyunsaturated fats are characterized by
the multiple double bonds.*

Classification of Fatty Acids by Length

Fatty acids are also classified by their length.

- <u>Short-chain</u> fatty acids have four to six carbon atoms. Short-chain fats are always saturated.
These fats are less likely to cause weight gain
than longer chain fatty acids due to the amount
of energy in each molecule. Short-chain fatty acids are said to contribute to the health of the immune system as well.

- <u>Medium-chain</u> fatty acids have eight to twelve carbon atoms and are found mostly in butterfat and the tropical oils. Like the short-chain fatty acids, these fats are absorbed directly and contribute to the health of the immune system.

- <u>Long-chain</u> fatty acids have from 14 to 18 carbon atoms and can be either saturated, monounsaturated or polyunsaturated. Stearic acid is an 18-carbon saturated fatty acid found chiefly in beef and mutton tallows. Oleic acid is an 18-carbon monounsaturated fat which is the chief component of olive oil. Another monounsaturated fatty acid is the 16-carbon palmitoleic acid which is found almost exclusively in animal fats.

- <u>Very-long-chain</u> fatty acids have 20 to 24 carbon atoms. They tend to be highly unsaturated, with four, five or six double bonds. In most cases, we either lack the enzymes to manufacture these molecules, or are very inefficient pathways. Therefore, we must obtain them from animal foods such as organ meats, egg yolks, butter and fish oils. The most well know of these are eicosapentaenoic acid (EPA) with 20 carbons and five double bonds; and docosahexaenoic acid (DHA) with 22 carbons and six double bonds which are found in fish oils.

As mentioned previously, the way in which a fatty acid is named is determined by the location of the

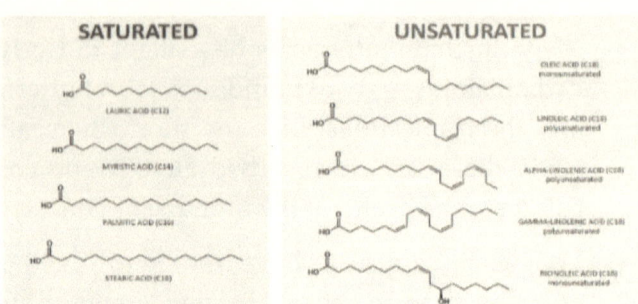

Figure 4: Saturated fatty and polyunsaturated fatty acid. Polyunsaturated fats differ by the number of carbon atoms as well as the number of double bonds.

first double bond (counted from the omega (ω-) or the n- end). <u>Omega-3 fatty acids</u> (or *n*-3 fatty acids) are polyunsaturated fatty acids (PUFAs) with a double bond at the third carbon atom from the end of the carbon chain. The three types of omega-3 fatty acids involved in human metabolism are α-linolenic acid (ALA) (found in plant oils), eicosapentaenoic acid (EPA), and docosahexaenoic acid (DHA) (both commonly found in marine oils). Common sources of plant oils containing the omega-3 ALA fatty acid include walnut, edible seeds, flaxseed oil. Sources of animal omega-3 EPA and DHA fatty acids include fish oils, egg oil, squid oils, and krill oil.

	Saturated Fatty Acid	Polyunsaturated Fatty Acid	Monounsaturated Fatty Acid
Canola	6	36	58
Safflower Oil	9	78	13
Sunflower Oil	11	69	20
Avocado Oil	12	14	74
Corn Oil	13	62	25
Olive Oil	15	11	73
Soybean Oil	15	62	24
Peanut Oil	18	34	48
Cottonseed Oil	27	54	19
Lard	41	12	47
Palm Oil	51	10	39
Beef Tallow	52	2	44
Butter Fat	66	4	30
Coconut Oil	92	2	6

Figure 5: Percentage of saturated, polyunsaturated and monounsaturated fat in cooking oils.

Fatty Acid Isomers

There is reference everywhere we turn to "trans" fats. And rightly so. These polyunsaturated fats are implicated in coronary artery disease, cancer, Alzheimer's, diabetes, depression, obesity, liver dysfunction and infertility. Most trans fats are the result of partial hydrogenation of vegetable oils to form a semisolid product to replace butter and other animal products. A quick look at a label that includes "partially hydrogenated" vegetable oil is going to have some trans fats even if the label says "zero trans fats". This is because FDA regulations states "Food manufacturers are allowed to list amounts of trans fat with less than 0.5 gram (1/2 g) per serving as

0 (zero) on the Nutrition Facts panel.

The position of the double bond determines the isomeric form of the molecule. If the hydrogen atoms are on the same side of the double bonds of the carbon chain it is in the _cis_ configuration (from the Latin, "on the same side"). This is the natural conformation and is the form recognized by the metabolic pathways in the cell. However, partial hydrogenation changes the double bonds that do not become chemically saturated, by twisting them so that the hydrogen atoms end up on different sides of the chain. This type of configuration is called _trans_, (from the Latin "across").

So, a molecule can be either a _trans_ or a _cis_ fatty acid depending on the configuration of the double bond. The configuration has implications for the physical-chemical properties of the molecule. The _trans_ configuration is straighter, while the _cis_ configuration is noticeably kinked. This three dimensionality of the molecule is important for the proper function of enzymes.

Eicosanoids

An eicosanoid is a hormone like molecules derived from arachidonic acid. The principle function of the eicosanoids is to signal specific biological activities. The term "eicosanoid" is derived from the Greek word "eikos", meaning twenty, because they are all derivatives of 20 carbon fatty acids. The eicosanoids include prostaglandins, leukotrienes, and thromboxane.

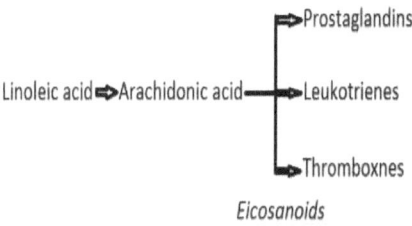

Figure 6: Formation of Eicosanoids.

Arachidonic acid is a unsaturated fatty acid, $C_{20}H_{32}O_2$, and a precursor in the biosynthesis of prostaglandins. This n-6 polyunsaturated fatty acid gives rise to the eicosanoid family of inflammatory mediators (prostaglandins, leukotrienes and related metabolites). The eicosanoids regulate the activities of inflammatory cells through the production of cytokines. We will ex-

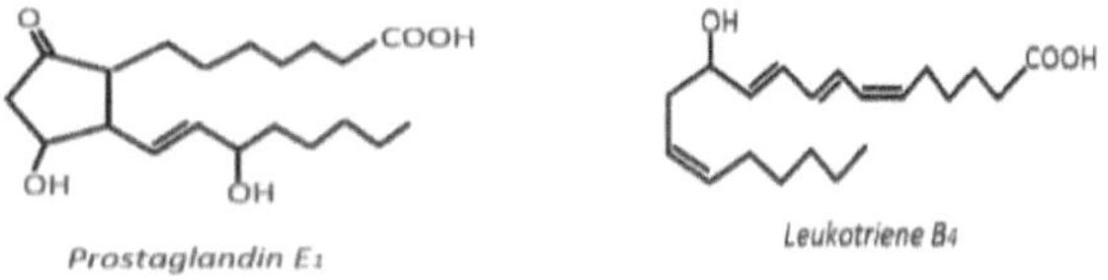

Figure 7: Structure of two eicosanoids from the prostaglandin and leukotriene families.

plore this effect later. Prostaglandins, leukotrienes and thromboxane regulate, blood clotting, inflammatory response, reproductive system, gastrointestinal tract, kidneys, and the respiratory tract.

2. Seed Oils

The typical Western diet contains 20 to 25-fold more n-6 fats than n-3 fats! This overabundance of n-6 fat is due to the high concentration of linoleic acid which is present in vegetable oils such as soy, corn, safflower, and sunflower. By contrast, there is a low intake of n-3 α-linolenic acid, which is present in leafy green vegetable.

Modern Western diets have omega-6/omega-3 ratios of approximately 30:9, although they can be as high as 50:10. And we know that vegetable oils are high in n-6 fatty acids. Corn oil has an n-6 to n-3 ratio of 58:1. Cotton seed oil is a close second at 54:1; soy bean at 50:7; and peanut at 32:0 (Figure 8).

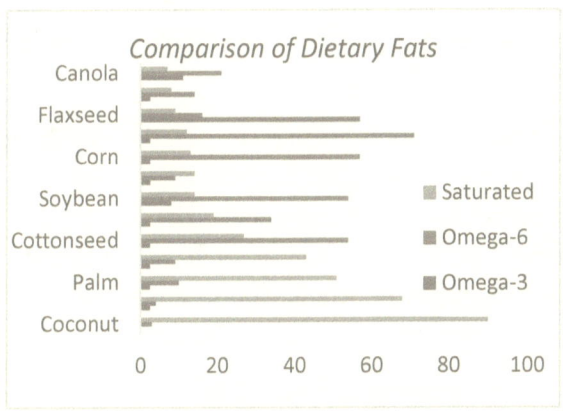

Figure 8: Comparison of the degree of unsaturation in dietary fats.

The term "vegetable oil" is a misnomer, a term created by marketing firms to promote these cooking oils. The fact is these are seed-derived oils. Civilizations began utilizing cooking oils thousands of years ago. Early populations used either the sun, or other fire heat source to heat whatever food stuffs they had available until the plants exuded oil that could be collected. In fact, Asian cultures such as Japan and China produced soy bean oil as early as 2000 B.C. Olive oil can be traced back to 3000 B.C. In North and Central America, peanuts and sunflower seeds were roasted and beaten into a paste before being boiled in water. The oil that rose to the surface was then skimmed off. Africans beat palm kernels and coconut meat which was then boiled, skimming the hot oil off the water.

Refinements to the extraction process were made over time. In the 1600s, a stamper press was used until the 1800s when John Smeaton invented the roll mill. In 1876, V.D. Anderson invented an improved screw press he termed *Expeller* which is a trade name that persists today.

Enhancements in pressing seeds were followed by improvements in extracting the oil. In 1856, Deiss obtained the first patent for extraction of oil using solvents. Petroleum derived solvents such as benzene were pumped through the material and collected. The benzene was removed resulting in extracted oil.

Most commercially available seed oils have only become available recently, as extraction technology has improved. Corn oil first became available in the 1960s. Cotton oil, the basis of Crisco, is an example of ways to make use of seeds that were, until recently, considered waste.

Vegetable oils comes from various parts of plants, in most cases from seeds (including sunflower, palm kernel, safflower, corn, cotton, sesame, canola, and grapeseed oils) or nuts (including peanut, soybean, almond, and walnut oils). A few special cases involve merely squeezing the oil from the flesh of the fruit of the plant. For example, coconut oil comes from the coconut's white meat, palm oil from the pulp of the palm fruit, and olive oil, as well as avocado, from the flesh.

The Manufacturing Process

While some oils, such as olive, avocado, and coconut are cold-pressed; seed oils are not suitable for cold pressing. These oils undergo multiple steps to produce a bland, clear, and consistent oil.

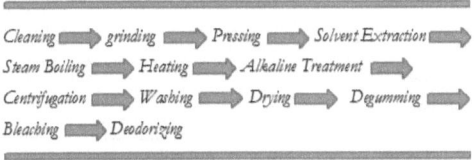

Cleaning and grinding:

- Seeds are passed over magnets to remove any trace metal before being deshelled. In the case of cotton, the seeds must be stripped of their lint as well as deshelled. In the case of corn, the kernel must undergo milling to separate the germ.

- The stripped seeds are then ground into coarse meal. Rollers crush the material to the proper consistency. The meal is heated to facilitate the extraction of the oil.

Pressing:

- The heated meal is then fed into a screw press, which increases the pressure progressively.

- Soybeans are usually not pressed at all before solvent extraction, because they have relatively little oil.

- The oil cake remaining in the press is processed by solvent extraction to attain the maximum yield. A volatile solvent (usually hexane) dissolves the oil out of the oil cake.

Removing solvent traces:

- The oil is recovered by distilling the hexane out.

- Ninety percent (95%) of the solvent remaining in the extracted oil simply evaporates, and collected for reuse.

- The rest is retrieved with the use of a stripping column.

- The oil is boiled by steam, and the lighter hexane floats upward.

Refining the oil:

- The oil is next refined to remove color, odor, and bitterness. Refining consists of heating the oil to between 107^0 and 188^0F, and mixing it with an alkaline substance such as sodium hydroxide or sodium carbonate.

- Soap forms from the reaction with the sodium hydroxide or sodium carbonate and removed by centrifuge.

- The oil is further washed to remove traces of soap and then dried.

- The oil is degummed by treating it with water heated to between 188^0 and 206^0F. The gums precipitate out and the dregs are removed by centrifuge.

- Oil is bleached by filtering it through activated charcoal, or activated clays that absorb certain pigmented material from the oil.

- The oil is then deodorized with steam in a vacuum at between 440^0 and 485^0F allowing the volatile taste and odor components to distill from the oil.

- Typically, citric acid at 0.01% is also added to the oil after deodorization to inactivate trace metals that might promote further oxidation.

History of the Vegetable Oil Hydrogenation Process

Hydrogenation is an important development which allows for the selective manipulation of the physical and chemical properties of cooking oils. Hydrogenation reduces the number of double bonds between carbon atoms in unsaturated fatty acids through the insertion of hydrogen molecules in the position the double bond occupies.

Liquid-phase hydrogenation was patented by William Normann in 1903 for the hydrogenation of liquid oils. In Normann's hydrogenation, the process converted vegetable oils, such as cotton seed oil, and also animal oils such as whale oil and fish into hard, white fats so that they could be used as lard substitute for making margarine.

William Proctor, a candle maker by trade joined with his brother-in-law, James Gamble, a soap-maker to compete with fourteen other soap and candle makers in Cincinnati, Ohio. In the 1890's, P&G gained control of the cottonseed oil business largely because of the monopoly by the meat-packers who controlled the price of lard and tallow needed to make candles and soap,. By 1905, they owned eight cottonseed mills in Mississippi. In 1907, P&G learning of Normann's hydrogenation process, P&G developed a solid that resembled lard.

Because rural electrification was forcing the candle business into obscurity, P&G looked for other markets for their new product. Since hydrogenated cottonseed oil resembled lard, why not introduce it as a food!

The new product was initially named Krispo, but trademark complications forced P&G to eventually chose Crisco, derived from CRYStalized Cottonseed Oil. In 1911, the Procter & Gamble Company launched their commercial production of hydrogenated cottonseed oil, and by the late 1970s roughly 60% of all edible oils and fats in the US were partially hydrogenated.

History of Margarine

Emperor Napoleon III took great interest in finding a cheap butter substitute to conform as closely as possible to butter's physical and chemical characteristics. Thus, the first margarine was invented in France by the French chemist, Hippolyte Mège-Mouriès in 1869 as part of a contest sponsored by the Emperor. Mège-Mouriès patented his process for churning beef tallow with milk to create an acceptable butter substitute.

While Mège-Mouriès margarine was cheap, his early variants were not very flavorful. Nor very appetizing. Early margarines were white and an attempt was made to add yellow dye to the product to give it the appearance of butter. However, American dairy farmers successfully lobbied for restrictions which banned the use of yellow dyes. By 1900, artificially colored butter was band in 30 U.S. states.

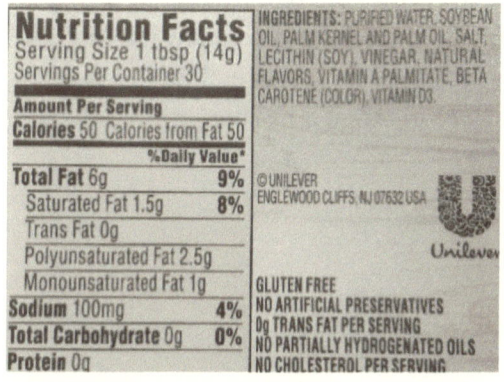

Figure 9: Typical margarine label.

In the 19th century, there began a movement in both Europe and the United States to migrate from the farm to the city. This movement meant the abandonment of the tradition of making butter and a push for the development of a butter substitute.

In 1923 Congress passed the pure foods and Drugs act which made it illegal to add any other ingredients to butter, even additives that would help make the butter more spreadable. But margarines could modify their products to meet the demands of the marketplace. Margarine's popularity skyrocketed.

Over time, vegetable oils such as cottonseed and soybean oils replaced the animal fats, and by World War I margarine was almost exclusively made from these vegetable oils. Butter scarcity during both World Wars, forced consumers to switch to margarine. And with the repeal of the margarine tax in 1950, the market continued to grow as individual states reversed their bans on colored margarine.

Today's margarines are manufactured from animal and vegetable fats, mixed with skim milk, salt, and emulsifiers. Margarines and vegetable fat spreads found in the market can range anywhere from 10 to 90% fat.

3. Lipid Peroxidation

Have you ever noticed the brown varnish-like gunk that form on the side of your pan after frying with vegetable oil? Ever wonder what was in it and what it was doing to you once consumed? This is the result of the heating of unstable polyunsaturated oil, undergoing a process called *polymerization*. Polymerization is the chemical process where individual fatty acids link together to form long chains. Linoleic fatty acid in polyunsaturated oils starts the chain reaction which continues forming the gunk that condenses on the side of pans, grill, etc. Linoleic fatty acid comprises 30 percent of peanut oil, 52 percent of soybean oil, and 60 percent of corn oil. It also degrades into other oxidation products such as free radicals, degraded fats, and oxidation products.

According to one analysis, a total of 130 volatile compounds were isolated from a piece of fried chicken alone!

While it is beyond the scope of this book to analyze all potentially toxic end products resulting from the exposure of polyunsaturated oils to oxygen, we will analyze the major breakdown products. In subsequent chapters we will explore the health implications, which are many. Lipid peroxidation is involved in various and numerous pathological states including inflammation, atherosclerosis, neurodegenerative diseases, and cancer.

Reactive Oxygen Species (ROS) is a phrase used to describe a number of reactive molecules and free radicals derived from oxygen. In general, harmful effects of reactive oxygen species on the cell are most often:

1. damage of DNA

2. oxidations of polyunsaturated fatty acids in lipids (lipid peroxidation)

3. oxidations of amino acids in proteins

4. oxidative deactivation of specific enzymes.

In particular, there are two prevalent ROS that profoundly affect lipids: hydroxyl radical (HO·) and hydroperoxyl (HO·2). The hydroxyl radical is chemically the most reactive species of activated oxygen. Enzymes in the cell, such as superoxide dismutase (SOD) moderates the damaging effects by converting these compounds into oxygen and water. However, this conversion is not always efficient, and residual peroxides persist in the cell. A cell produces around 50 hydroxyl radicals every second. In a full day, each cell would generate 4 million hydroxyl radicals, which are either neutralized, or live on to attack other biomolecules. While ROS are produced as a product of normal cellular functioning, excessive amounts, can overwhelm the cellular defenses, and cause deleterious effects.

Lipid peroxidation is a degradation process involving the double bond(s) found in both mono and polyunsaturated fatty acids, causing a deterioration of food quality (odor, flavor, color, texture, toxicity). This is collectively known as turning *rancid*. The well-known targets of damaging and potentially lethal peroxidative modification are glycolipids, phospholipids (PLs), and cholesterol (Ch).

The overall process of lipid peroxidation consists of multiple steps where hydroxyl radical interacts with the polyunsaturated fatty acid (Figure 10). Once lipid peroxidation is started, a chain reaction continues until termination products are produced.

Lipid peroxidation of unsaturated fatty acids produces a wide variety of oxidation products. The main primary products of lipid peroxidation are lipid hydroperoxides (LOOH). Among the many different aldehydes which can be formed as secondary products during lipid peroxidation, malondialdehyde (MDA), propanal, hexanal, and 4-hydroxynonenal (4-HNE) have been extensively studied. MDA appears to be the most mutagenic product of lipid peroxidation, whereas 4-HNE is the most toxic.

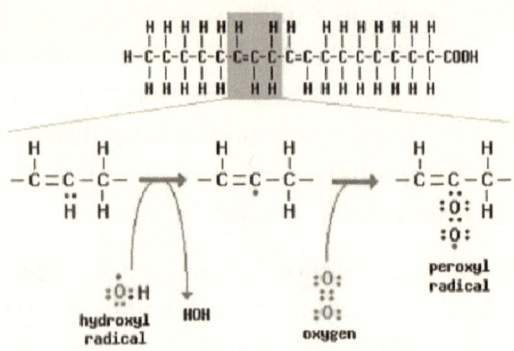

Figure 10: Lipid peroxidation reaction. A common target for peroxidation are the unsaturated fats in cellular membranes.

Lipid peroxidation is not limited to the cellular environment. During the frying process, cooking oil is exposed to an extremely high temperature in the presence of air and moisture. Under such conditions, a complex series of chemical reactions takes place. Repeatedly heating the cooking oils initiates a series of chemical reactions, modifying the fat constituents of cooking oil through oxidation, hydrolysis, polymerization, and isomerization, eventually resulting in lipid peroxidation. Lipid peroxidation generates a wide spectrum of volatile or non-volatile components, including free fatty acids, alcohols, aldehydes, ketones, hydrocarbons, *trans* isomers, cyclic and epoxy compounds. These toxic products are absorbed by the food, and eventually into the gastrointestinal tract and thereafter enter the systemic circulation.

<u>Malondialdehyde</u> (MDA) is a highly reactive three carbon di-aldehyde produced as a byproduct of polyunsaturated fatty acid peroxidation and arachidonic acid metabolism. MDA readily combines with several functional groups on molecules including proteins, lipoproteins, and DNA. Malondialdehyde is a biomarker of lipid peroxidation that has been widely associated with food rancidity as well as many human diseases.

<u>4-Hydroxynonenal</u> (4-HNE), is the major end product generated by decomposition of arachidonic acid and larger polyunsaturated fatty acids, through enzymatic or non-enzymatic processes. It is generally accepted that 4-HNE is derived from the decomposition of n-6 polyunsaturated fatty acids at the n-2 position by hydroperoxide. Therefore, phospholipids containing linoleic acid (LA, 18:2, n-6) and arachidonic acid (AA, 20:4, n-6) on cytoplasmic membranes or n-6 polyunsaturated fatty acids which are abundant in vegetable oils are considered the major source for 4-HNE production. 4-HNE is an extraordinarily reactive compound. 4-HNE is the most intensively studied lipid peroxidation end-product, in relation to its cytotoxic role inhibiting gene expression and promoting the development and progression of different diseases.

Other compounds that are created in vegetable oils during processing are monochlorpropane-diols and glycidol esters (MCPDs). 3-monochloropropane-1,2-

diol (3-MCPD) is a contaminant which occurs through food processing. It is formed in foods containing fat and salt when they are exposed to high temperatures during production. The formation of 3-MCPD in food is influenced by many factors, including temperature, pH, moisture content, sugar and lipid content. It is registered at the federal level as a <u>rodenticide</u> with restricted use, under the name α-chlorohydrin!

According to the European Food Safety Authority, studies have linked 3-MCPD with infertility in rats, suppression of the immune function and possible carcinogenicity. In December 2007, the presence of fatty esters of 3-MCPD (3-MCPD esters) was reported for the first time in a number of foodstuffs including refined edible fats, such as margarine and oils, as well as infant formula and breast milk. While there are a number of toxicological animal studies on 3-MCPD, little is known about the occurrence, toxicokinetic profile, or toxicity of 3-MCPD esters.

In September 2010, the California Environmental Protection Agency issued a 30-page report on the "Evidence on the Carcinogenicity of 3-Monochloropropane-1,2-diol (3-MCPD; α-Chlorohydrin). The findings summarize that:

Kidney Tumors

- "3-MCPD significantly increased the incidence of malignant, and benign and malignant kidney tumors in male Sprague-Dawley rats. Tumors appeared early. Kidney tumors are rare in untreated male Sprague-Dawley rats.

- Combined benign and malignant kidney tumors were significantly increased in treated female Sprague-Dawley rats. Kidney tumors are rare in untreated female Sprague-Dawley rats.
- Benign kidney tumors were increased in treated male Fischer rats.
- Benign kidney tumors were increased in treated female Fischer rats.
- 3-MCPD increased renal tubular hyperplasia in both sexes and strains.
- 3-MCPD exacerbated chronic progressive nephropathy in both sexes and strains.

Mammary Tumors

- 3-MCPD significantly increased the incidence of benign and malignant mammary tumors in male Fischer rats.
- 3-MCPD increased glandular hyperplasia of the mammary gland in male Fischer rats.
- Mammary gland tumors are uncommon in male Fischer rats.

Leydig cell tumors

- 3-MCPD significantly increased the incidence of benign and malignant Leydig cell tumors in male Fischer rats.
- 3-MCPD significantly increased the incidence of Leydig cell tumors in male Sprague-Dawley rats.

- Leydig cell tumors are uncommon in Sprague-Dawley rats."

Polymers and Cyclic fatty acid monomers (CFAM) are potentially toxic, and the latter are detected at levels 0.01-0.7% in used frying oils. Cyclic monomers derived from polyunsaturated fatty acids have been reported to elicit toxic responses when fed to laboratory animals at low dietary levels. However, studies in CFAMs are scarce. When CFAM were administered orally to mice, a higher death rate was observed. Weight gain in weaning rats was decreased and the liver weight and death rate increased in rat pups from mothers fed CFAM. CFAM feeding also reduced the number of pups per litter. CFAM are also incorporated into cultured heart cells where they alter the electrophysiological properties.

Cooking fumes, especially from frying, contain several specific agents which may give adverse health effects in the lung. Studies by Sjaastad and Svendsen have shown that cooking fumes contain aldehydes such as formaldehyde, acetaldehyde and acrolein. Acrolein and aldehydes are toxic and strong irritants for the skin, eyes, and nasal passages.

4. Atherosclerosis and Cardiovascular Disease

Heart disease was for the most part unknown in 1900. In fact, the first journal publication on heart disease did not appear until 1921. Since then, heart disease has increased from 1,000 people in 1910 to 58.5 million in 2005; an increase of 5,820% (Figure 11). Coincidentally, Proctor and Gamble introduced Mazola corn

oil and Crisco in 1911. Prior to 1911, the primary cooking fats were saturated fats from butter and tallow.

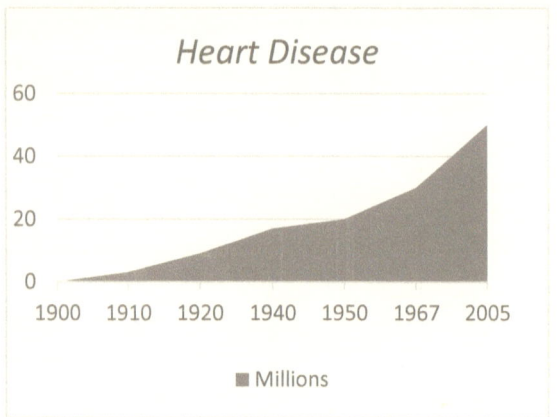

*Figure 11: Number of People Diagnoses with Heart Dis-
ease 1900 to 2005. Crisco and corn oil were introduced in
1911.*

While we are better able to treat heart disease,
the prevalence continues to rise. Cardiovascular disease
(CVD) is one of the leading major causes of morbidity
and mortality worldwide.

By 1950, coronary heart disease, was the leading
cause of death in the United States, responsible for more
than 30% of all deaths. Myocardial infarction (MI)
caused no more than three thousand deaths per year in
1930. By 1960, there were at least 500,000 MI deaths per
year in the US (Figure 12).

During that time, research began to solidify
around the *cholesterol hypothesis* as the cause of heart disease. To better understand the cholesterol hypothesis,

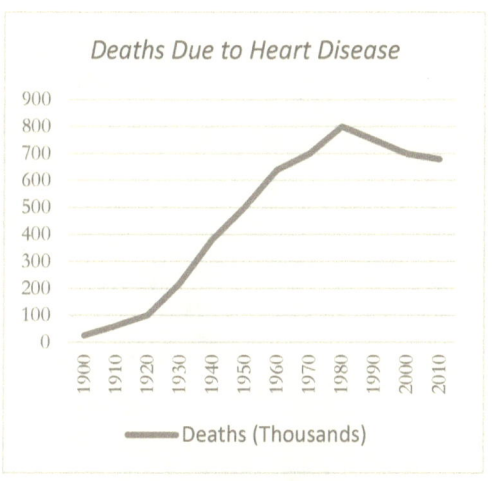

Figure 12: Deaths (In Thousands) Due to Heart Disease.

we need to review the data and assumptions behind it. The hypothesis argues that cholesterol in the blood is deposited in the arteries thereby causing the blockage seen in atherosclerosis. The first published evidence for the cholesterol hypothesis came when German researcher Windaus who noted that aortas of patients with atherosclerosis contain more cholesterol in their aortas compared to healthy individuals.

The landmark study came in 1913, when Nikolaj Nikolajewitsch Anitschkow fed cholesterol to rabbits causing atherosclerosis. In subsequent work, Anitschkow concluded that the process of atherosclerosis starts with the formation of fatty streaks. However, cholesterol is only soluble in oil so many of these studies used corn oil as the vehicle for administration thereby putting the results in question.

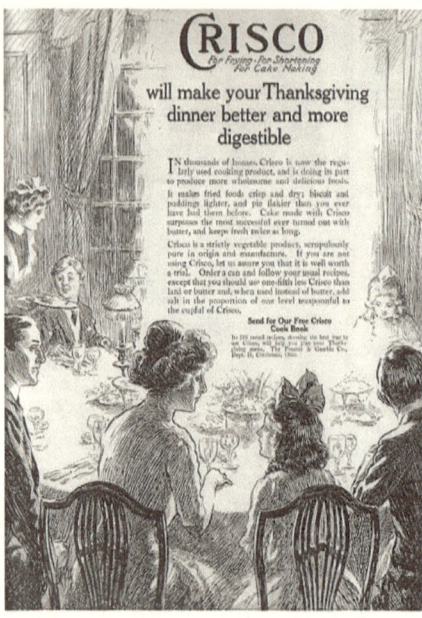

Figure 13: Crisco advertisement November 1912 from the Ladies Home Journal.

Around the same time, the seed oil industry was in crisis. Seed oils were being used in paints and plastics but were being displaced by petroleum based products. The industry needed new markets, and proposed a marketing strategy that "vegetable" oils were healthier than traditional animal fats. After all, polyunsaturated fats were observed to lower cholesterol blood levels. Crisco, initially made with hydrogenated cottonseed oil, is the quintessential imitation food. Crisco advertisements from the 1900 frequently included health claims. Procter & Gamble's first ad campaign introduced the "all-vegetable" shortening as "a healthier alternative to cooking with animal fats." An ad in 1912 claimed "It's digestible" (Figure 13). Crisco was made by hydrogenating cottonseed oil to make a product the resembled lard. Unfortunately, hydrogenation introduces trans fats, the consequences of which were not know at the time.

In 1939, Muller published findings in the *Annals*

of Internal Medicine that patients with familial cases of hypercholesterolemia had significantly more cardiovascular disease than people without increased plasma cholesterol levels, thereby confirming Anitschkow's earlier work postulating cholesterol is a causal factor in atherosclerosis.

This was the beginning of many studies that supported the cholesterol hypothesis. A 1955 report on artery plaques in soldiers killed during the Korean War received a significant amount of attention. Postmortem examination of remains showed significant development of atherosclerosis despite their young age. They concluded dietary influence had caused early development of atherosclerotic plaques. There were other epidemiological studies showing that Japanese had almost as much pathogenic plaque despite having less animal fats in their diet but these were mostly ignored.

The American Heart Association (AHA) was a relatively obscure association until Procter & Gamble gave $1.5 million to the radio show, *Truth or Consequences*, allowing the organization to go national. The AHA aired a fund raiser in 1956 on all three major networks promoting the *prudent Diet*. The panel included renowned researchers at the time and supported the *cholesterol hypothesis* as the cause of the heart disease. However, they went one step further proposing a diet of corn oil, margarine, chicken and cold cereal replacing butter, lard, beef and eggs. Dr. Dudley White, was the lone panelist who disputed his colleagues at the AHA. Dr. White reminded the panel that myocardial infarction was non-existent in 1900 when corn oil was unavailable and when egg consumption was three times what it was in 1956. Dr. White is quoted as having said: "I began my practice as a cardiologist in 1921 and I never saw an MI patent until 1928. Back in the MI free days before 1920, the fats were butter and lard and I think that we would all benefit from the kind of diet that we had at a time when no one had ever heard the words "corn oil."

This followed with the AHA issuing dietary guidelines in 1957. The 1957 AHA report concluded that there was a causal relationship between saturated fats and the pathogenesis of atherosclerosis.

The food industry quickly took up the banner promoting health benefits of vegetable oils. A Mazola oil ad from 1951 touted "no cholesterol". Another ad made such claims as: "Best for cutting down saturated fats in your diet"; "Polyunsaturates are a plus in Mazola"; "Take this ad to your doctor…" The ad goes on to claim a 17% reduction in serum cholesterol". A major medical journal advertisement recommended Fleishmann's unsalted margarine for patients with high blood pressure.

Ancel Keys, a professor at the University of Minnesota, published his Six Country Analysis in 1953. Keys suggested an association between dietary fat and mortality from heart disease. Critics pointed out that Keys had data for 22 countries, but selected data from just 6 (Keys excluded countries with a high fat diet and low rates of heart disease).

In 1977, the *Select Committee on Nutrition and Human Needs* of the United States Senate published a committee report titled *Dietary Goals for the United States*. The Committee, chaired by George McGovern, sought to "set national dietary goal for the country." The report was released with a press briefing including several prominent nutritional researchers including Dr. Beverly Winikoff (Rockefeller Foundation), Dr. Philip Lee (University of California), Dr. D.M. Hegsted (Harvard), and a handful of Senators. The Committee recommended:

- Increase carbohydrate intake between 55 - 60 percent of calories,

- Decrease dietary fat intake to no more than 30 percent of calories, with a reduction in intake of saturated fat, and recommended approximately equivalent distributions among saturated, polyunsaturated, and monounsaturated fats to meet the 30 percent target,

- Decrease cholesterol intake to 300 mg per day,

- Decrease sugar intake to 15 percent of calories,

- Decrease salt intake to 3 g per day.

The report was met with skepticism from both industry and research community who felt the literature at the time did not support the specific intake goals. Nonetheless, the Department of Agriculture and the Department of Health, Education, and Welfare established a joint committee whose goal was to focus on the controversy that existed among some nutritionists and others concerned with food, nutrition, and health. They collectively published the *Dietary Guidelines for Americans* brochure in February 1980.

At the same time, the FDA *Select Committee on GRAS Substances* (SCOGS) issued their opinion on Hydrogenated soybean oil. The GRAS (Generally Recognized As Safe) ingredient reviews were conducted by the Select Committee in response to a 1969 White House directive by then President Richard M. Nixon. The Select Committee found: "There is no evidence in the available information on hydrogenated soybean oil that demonstrates, or suggests reasonable grounds to suspect, a hazard to the public when it is used as a direct or indirect food ingredient at levels that are now current or that might reasonably be expected in the future." The Committee report was dismissive on the effect of transfats. The opinion concluded: "the weight of evidence indicates that trans-monoenoic acids, the principal geometric isomers present in hydrogenated soybean oil, are not hypercholesterolemic. Similarly, the results of animal experimentation indicate that trans-acids of hydrogenated soybean oil are not atherogenic at normal dietary levels." Of course, we now know that is not the case.

The same committee issued their GRAS opinion on coconut oil, peanut oil, and oleic acid in 1975. They found "no evidence in the available information on coconut oil, peanut oil, and oleic acid that demonstrates, or suggests reasonable grounds to suspect, a hazard to the public as they are now used in paper and cotton packaging material for food at levels now current or as they might reasonably be expected to be used for such purposes in the future." Clearly, the FDA did not differentiate between types of oil. They went on to conclude: "There is no evidence in the available information on linoleic acid that demonstrates, or suggests reasonable grounds to suspect, a hazard to the public when it is used as a nutrient or dietary supplement at levels now current or that might reasonably be expected in the future."

In 1968, Paul Leren published *The Effect of Plasma Cholesterol Lowering Diet in Male Survivors of Myocardial Infarction. A Controlled Clinical Trial.* This was the first long term study which supported a reduction in cardiovascular disease with a cholesterol lowering diet. In 1984, the *Lipid Research Clinics Coronary Primary Prevention Trial* results were published supporting the relationship of the incidence of coronary heart disease to lower cholesterol. This trial showed that cholestyramine, a drug which lowered plasma cholesterol by about 10%, lowered the relative risk of coronary heart disease by almost 20%. Then, in 1994, the well-known *Scandinavian Simvastatin Survival Study Group: Randomized Trial of Cholesterol Lowering in 4444 Patients with Coronary Heart Disease: The Scandinavian Simvastatin Survival Study (4S)* was published in the Lancet. In this study simvastatin (a statin drug) used to reduce plasma cholesterol levels, decreased levels by approximately 25% with a reduction in the relative risk of death due to coronary heart disease by 42%.

These studies served to firmly entrench the cholesterol hypothesis. While the American Medical Association initially did not support the hypothesis, the American Heart Association was firmly on board. And in 1961 the AHA advocated the substitution of polyunsaturated oils for saturated fats, despite little evidence to support this statement.

Cracks form in the Cholesterol Hypothesis

Cracks started to develop in the cholesterol hypothesis. In June 1966, Drs. Rose, Thomson, and Williams published an article in the British Medical Journal on the results of a prospective study of corn oil in patients with Ischemic Heart Disease. Patients were equally divided into one of three groups receiving either 80g/day corn oil, or olive oil; or a control group. Patients in both oil groups were instructed to avoid fried foods, fatty meat, sausages, pastry, ice-cream, cheese, cakes, etc. Milk, eggs, and butter were restricted. The oil supplement was divided into three equal doses at mealtimes. The patients were followed for two years. The patients receiving corn oil had a significant reduction in total cholesterol, but shockingly had 25% more deaths than either the olive oil or control group! The proportions of patients remaining alive and free of re-infarction (fatal or non-fatal) was greater for the control group (75%)than for the two oil groups (olive oil 57%, corn oil 52%).

from 1995–1997, and were followed-up on cause-specific mortality for 10 years (510,97 person-years in total). The authors concluded that "public health recommendations regarding the 'dangers' of cholesterol should be revised. This is especially true for women, for whom moderately elevated cholesterol (by current standards) may prove to be not only harmless but even beneficial."

K. Anderson *et al.*, examined the relationship of cholesterol and mortality based on 30 Years of follow-up from the Framingham Study. From 1951 to 1955 serum cholesterol levels were measured in 1,959 men and 2,415 women aged between 31 and 65 years who were free of cardiovascular disease (CVD) and cancer. They found that under age 50 years, cholesterol levels are directly related with 30-year overall and CVD mortality. However, after age 50 years there is no increased overall mortality with either high or low serum cholesterol levels!

In 2012, Saremi *et al.*, published an association with frequent statin use and an accelerated progression of coronary artery calcification in a study of 197 diabetic patients without previous coronary artery disease. The frequent statin users had significantly lower, and nearly optimal, LDL-cholesterol levels. Yet, despite the lowering of cholesterol levels, the use of statins was associated with an acceleration of calcific atherosclerosis.

Other randomized controlled trials in largely nondiabetic populations, with no previous coronary ar-

And remember the *Prudent Diet* of corn oil, margarine, fish, chicken and cold cereal promoted on national television? The results were published in 1966 in the *Journal of the American Medical Association.* The diet group, had an average serum cholesterol of 220 mg/dl, compared to 250 mg/dl in the meat-and-potatoes control group. However, there were eight deaths from heart disease among the Prudent Diet group, and none among those who ate meat three times a day. (Dr. Jolliffe the lead author died in 1961 from a vascular thrombosis.)

In 1987, Anderson, Castelli, and Levy, published the "Cholesterol and Mortality: 30 Years of Follow-up from the Framingham Study" in the Journal of the American Medical Association. The Framingham study is a long-term study that looked at serum cholesterol levels in 1,959 men and 2,415 women from 1951 to 1955. The individuals were between 31 – 65 years and free of cardiovascular disease. The authors found that after age 50 years of age, there is no increased overall mortality with either high or low serum cholesterol levels.

Harcombe *et al.* conducted a systemic review and meta-analysis of reports, published prior to 1983, which examined the relationship between dietary fat, serum cholesterol and the development of heart disease that may have been used to support the dietary fat guidelines of 1977 and 1983. The dietary fat guidelines were released by the US (1977) and UK (1983) governments to significantly reduce saturated fat consumption. Shockingly, the authors concluded that evidence from randomized controlled trials **did not** support the recommendations introduced in the dietary fat guidelines! They concluded that "dietary recommendations were introduced for 220 million US and 56 million UK citizens by 1983, in the absence of supporting evidence from RCTs" (Random Controlled Trials). Data from six (6) clinical studies of men with coronary heart-disease had blood-cholesterol lower than the expected values!

The Honolulu Heart Program looked at cholesterol concentrations in 3,572 Japanese/American men (aged 71–93 years). They compared changes in cholesterol levels over 20 years to all-cause mortality. Mean cholesterol fell significantly with increasing age, and those individuals with low cholesterol had an increase in the number of deaths. This casts doubt on the recommendation of lowering cholesterol levels, especially in the elderly.

Research published in March 1993 showed that heart disease worsened in those who switched from butter to polyunsaturated-rich margarine. The study compared 85,000 women who ate polyunsaturated margarine, to those who did not consume margarine. Those who ate four (4) or more teaspoons of polyunsaturated margarine a day had a sixty-six (66%) percent *increased* risk of Coronary Heart Disease (CHD). A similar review of men in the Framingham Study published in 1995 also found that six (6) teaspoons a day increased risk by nearly a third. The authors conclude: "Intake of margarine may predispose to development of CHD in men".

In 1996, an article was published in the Israel

Journal of Medical Science titled: *Diet and disease--the Israeli paradox: possible dangers of a high omega-6 polyunsaturated fatty acid diet*. The authors state that "Israel has one of the highest dietary polyunsaturated/saturated fat ratios in the world; the consumption of omega-6 polyunsaturated fatty acids (PUFA) is about 8% higher than in the USA, and 10-12% higher than in most European countries." They conclude that "despite such national habits, there is paradoxically a high prevalence of cardiovascular diseases, hypertension, non-insulin-dependent diabetes mellitus and obesity; all diseases that are associated with hyperinsulinemia (HI) and insulin resistance (IR), and grouped together as the insulin resistance syndrome or syndrome X. There is also an increased cancer incidence and mortality rate, especially in women, compared with western countries. Studies suggest that high omega-6 linoleic acid consumption might aggravate HI and IR, in addition to being a substrate for lipid peroxidation and free radical formation. Thus, rather than being beneficial, high omega-6 PUFA diets may have some long-term side effects, within the cluster of hyperinsulinemia, atherosclerosis and tumorigenesis."

It has been known since 1994 that intake of polyunsaturated fats affects the fatty-acid content of aortic plaques. Felton *et al.* compared the fatty-acid composition of aortic plaques with that of post-mortem serum and adipose tissue. They found a positive association between serum and adipose omega-3, omega-6 polyunsaturated fatty acids as well as monounsaturated fatty acids, with plaque formation. No associations were found with saturated fatty acids. These findings imply a direct influence of dietary polyunsaturated fatty acids on aortic plaque formation.

An article in the journal *Annals of Internal Medicine*, published in 2003 identified 72 studies: 45 cohort studies and 27 randomized controlled trials looking at the association between dietary fatty acid intake and coronary disease' The 32 cohort studies included 530,525 people. When comparing the top third to those in the bottom third of dietary fatty acid intake, only trans fatty acid intake was significantly associated with a risk of coronary disease. This comprehensive review found no evidence that saturated fat increases the risk of coronary disease, or that polyunsaturated fats have a cardio protective effect, in contrast to current recommendations! Since then numerous meta-analysis of prospective epidemiologic studies have concluded the same; that there is no significant evidence for concluding that dietary saturated fat is associated with an increased risk of coronary heart disease or cardiovascular disease.

Even the American Heart Association has backed away from their long-held recommendation of reducing dietary cholesterol. "As anticipated, the panel did not include a recommendation for dietary cholesterol, agreeing with an American Heart Association/American College of Cardiology report that concluded there isn't scientific evidence to show it reduces the artery-clogging LDL cholesterol in the blood. In the

2010 Dietary Guidelines, Americans were told to limit dietary cholesterol to 300 mg a day."

Galvao *et al.*, in 2012 compared a standard low-fat diet to high-fat diets enriched with either saturated fat (palmitate and stearate) or PUFA (linoleic and α-linolenic acids) in hamsters with genetic cardiomyopathy. Their results show that a high intake of saturated fat improves survival in heart failure compared with a high PUFA diet or low-fat diet. They also found an increase in mitochondrial permeability in the PUFA group. This confirmed the work of Galvao *et al.* from the previous year, showing that heart failure hamsters fed a diet high in saturated fat showed increased survival compared with hamsters fed a diet high in PUFA or the control standard diet.

In 2013, the results of the Sydney Diet Heart Study were published. The study, titled: *Use of Dietary Linoleic Acid for Secondary Prevention of Coronary Heart Disease and Death,* looked at the effectiveness of replacing dietary saturated fat with omega 6 linoleic acid, for prevention of coronary heart disease and death. Participants were 458 men aged 30-59 years with a recent coronary event. They replaced dietary saturated fats with omega-6 linoleic acid (from safflower oil and safflower oil polyunsaturated margarine). Controls received no specific dietary instruction or study foods. The ssubstitution of dietary linoleic acid in place of saturated fats increased the rate of death from all causes, coronary heart disease, and cardiovascular disease.

41

Despite the overwhelming evidence to the contrary, the American College of Cardiology and American Heart Association continues to demonize saturated fats. Their 2013 guidelines on lifestyle management to reduce CVD risk omitted a target for total dietary fat but did recommend a goal of 5%-6% of calories from saturated fat.

The basis for their argument is the observation that polyunsaturated fats decrease levels of serum LDL-cholesterol, thereby reducing cardiovascular disease. Yet, this hypothesis is easily proven false. In a meta-analysis of over 60 trials, higher intakes of saturated fat were, as expected, associated with an increase in LDL-cholesterol levels. However, there was an increase in high-density lipoprotein cholesterol (HDL-C) as well, coupled with a decrease in triglyceride levels, for a net neutral effect on the ratio of total cholesterol to HDL cholesterol. Although saturated fats increase LDL-C, they reduce the LDL particle number. Total LDL particle number is considered a stronger indicator of CV risk than traditional cholesterol measures.

An updated meta-analysis of linoleic acid intervention trials showed no evidence of cardiovascular benefit. These studies suggest that a diet containing saturated fats is either neutral, or prolongs life compared with a diet high in polyunsaturated fat. Not only is there a lack of survival benefit with the high PUFA diet, but the high PUFA diet is associated with a 75% increase in plasma free fatty acids. Clinical studies in the 1960s found an association between elevated free fatty acids and ventricular arrhythmias. It was later shown that plasma fatty acid concentration is a strong predictor of sudden cardiac death. While it is possible that the elevation in free fatty acids triggers arrhythmias, there is further evidence that PUFA's are directly involved with the pathogenesis of atherosclerosis.

What is Cholesterol?

To better understand atherosclerosis, and the role polyunsaturated acid play in the development of heart disease, we need to have a basic understanding of the mechanisms involved. One often hears about the artery clogging effects of fats. Even the American Heart Association mentions "artery-clogging LDL cholesterol" in their literature. These are frequent seen in articles on atherosclerosis and usually followed with a discussion on the "good fats (polyunsaturated vegetable oil) and the "bad fats" (saturated fats). It is unfortunate that the scientific method has failed us and marketing strategies prevail over our understanding of the pathogenesis of this disease.

Cholesterol is a lipid molecule and is manufactured by all animal cells. It is a major structural molecule in cell walls, as well as a precursor for the biosynthesis of steroid hormones, bile acids, and vitamin D. Cholesterol is only slightly soluble in water. So, to enable cholesterol transport in the blood, cholesterol must be transported inside vesicles called lipoproteins. There are several types of lipoproteins found in the blood. In order of increasing density, they are chylomicrons, very-low-density lipoprotein (VLDL), low-density lipoprotein (LDL), intermediate-density lipoprotein (IDL), and high-density lipoprotein (HDL). So, when a physician

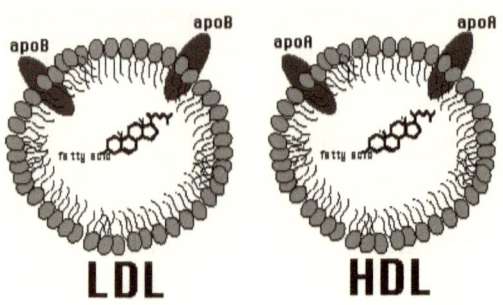

Figure 14: LDL and HDL lipoproteins. The LDL and HDL cholesterol particle are spherical globule with a lipoprotein - apo B is embedded in the matrix of the LDL particle.

orders a fractionated cholesterol panel, the results are just a profile of the different lipoproteins.

LDL particles are the major blood cholesterol carriers. Each one contains approximately 1,500 molecules of cholesterol. The LDL cholesterol particle is a spherical globule with a lipoprotein - apo B embedded in its matrix. The HDL particle is similar to the LDL lipoprotein except for the presence of apo A in its matrix (Figure 14).

Nature has developed this elegant means of transporting cholesterol around the body. As a cell senses the need for cholesterol, it produces apo B protein receptors on its cell membrane. The Apo B binds to the receptor protein and the LDL particle is released into the cell cytoplasm (Figure 15).

The reverse is true if a cell has too much choles-terol. The HDL particle transports excess cholesterol to the liver where it is recycled (Figure 16). Cholesterol lev-

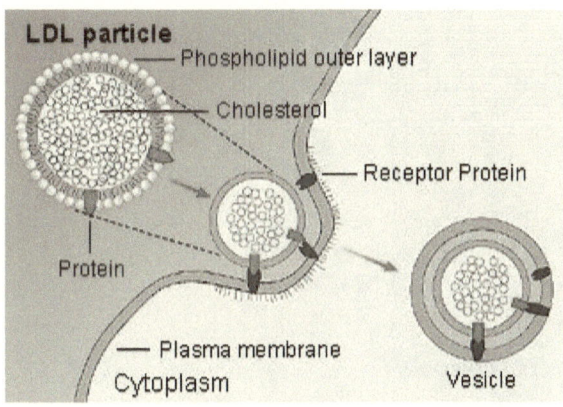

Figure 15: The LDL particle binds to Apo-B receptors on the cell membrane thereby releasing cholesterol into the cell.

els are tightly controlled and individual levels are "set" due to that person's genetic predisposition. In other words, as you consume more cholesterol, the liver re-duces the amount manufactured, as well as the corol-lary, the less you consume, the more is produced. Over-all, 90% of cholesterol is synthesized in the liver so die-tary cholesterol impact is negligible.

Familial hypercholesterolemia (High cholesterol **caused by a specific genetic defect**) is due to a defect in the LDL receptor that prevents the clearance of LDL particles from the circulation.

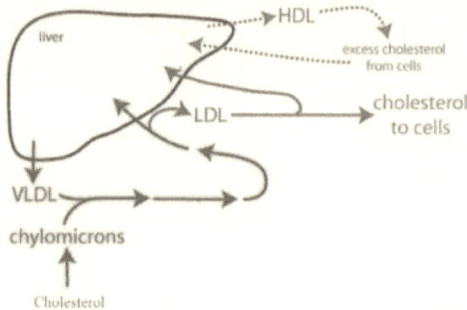

Figure 16: lipoproteins transport cholesterol to cells. Excess cholesterol is removed by HDL where it is returned to the liver for recycling. Dietary cholesterol is transported via chylomicrons either to the liver or eventually to LDL particles.

Atherosclerosis

Investigators began to notice in the 1980's that half of those who suffer coronary heart disease had LDL-cholesterol levels within normal limits. In the Women's Health Study, 46% of first cardiovascular events occurred in women with LDL cholesterol levels less than 130 mg/dl, the "desirable" target for primary prevention set by the National Cholesterol Education Program (NCEP). Castelli published a series of articles noting that more than 75 percent of patients with an acute coronary syndrome or a myocardial infarction had normal plasma values of cholesterol, LDL cholesterol and/or HDL cholesterol.

The protective effects of statins against cardiovascular disease as seen in the *Scandinavian Simvastatin Survival Study Group* did not stand up to challenges from other clinical studies. As with many studies showing decreases in plasma LDL cholesterol with statin administration, the protection against cardiovascular disease was simply not there. At least seven follow-on studies suggest that LDL-cholesterol blood level is unlikely to be an important causal factor for cardiovascular disease.

The clinical failure of the cholesterol lowering drug Vytorin in the ENHANCE Trial (The Effect of Combination Ezetimibe and High-Dose Simvastatin vs. Simvastatin Alone on the Atherosclerotic Process in Patients with Heterozygous Familial Hypercholesterolemia) is prompting a reexamination of the rational for using statins to treat atherosclerosis. Statins are sold by numerous pharmaceutical companies. Lovastatin (Mevacor) and simvastatin (Zocor); rosuvastatin (Crestor); pravastatin (Pravachol); fluvastatin (Lescol); and atorvastatin (Lipitor). Vytorin is a formulation that combines simvastatin with a non-statin cholesterol absorption blocker, ezetimibe (Zetia).

The ENHANCE trial showed a significant decrease in low-density lipoprotein cholesterol (LDL-C) levels over the two years of the study as expected. However, the intima-media thickness (IMT) in the arteries increased in both groups, but was significantly greater in the Vytorin group than in the simvastatin group! IMT is considered to be an important marker of atherosclerosis and a strong predictor of future myocardial infarction. In other words, the reduction in cholesterol levels did not make a difference in preventing atherosclerosis.

However, the combined effect of two cholesterol agents appeared to accelerate atherosclerosis in this study! The trial was eventually published in *New England Journal of Medicine* in April, 2008 after some delay.

The ENHANCE trial simply confirmed the findings that Abramson and Wright published in 2007. They conducted a meta-analysis of eight randomized controlled trials and concluded (1) total mortality is not reduced with statin therapy, (2) serious adverse events were not reduced either, and (3) the absolute frequency of cardiovascular events was reduced by only 1.5%! In other words, you would have to treat 67 patients with statins over a 5-year period for one patient to benefit (a 98.5% failure rate).

To be fair, not all statins are equal in their ability to reduce LDL-cholesterol. So, let's look at CRESTOR (rosuvastatin calcium) which is widely regarded to be one of the most potent statins. According to the FDA approved labeling, Crestor lowers LDL-cholesterol by an average of 55% after 12 weeks of dosing at 20mg per day.

As justification of approval, the label references the JUPITER study (In the Justification for the Use of Statins in Primary Prevention: An Intervention Trial Evaluating Rosuvastatin). "The effect of CRESTOR (rosuvastatin calcium) on the occurrence of major cardiovascular (CV) disease events was assessed in 17,802 men (≥ 50 years) and women (≥ 60 years) who had no clinically evident cardiovascular disease...)". "Study participants had a median baseline LDL-C of 108 mg/dl.

Study participants were randomly assigned to placebo (n=8,901) or rosuvastatin 20 mg once daily (n=8,901) and were followed for a mean duration of 2 years. Rosuvastatin reduced the risk of major CV events with an absolute risk reduction of just 1.2%!

In other words, the absolute risk reduction of having a major cardiovascular event after taking Crestor for two years is in line with the meta-analysis of the other statin trials. This is hardly a ringing endorsement of the cholesterol hypothesis.

In a large clinical study involving over 10,000 participants who were randomly assigned to two groups for comparison; those using very high dose Lipitor (80mg) achieved markedly lower LDL-C levels compared to those using a much lower dose of Pravastatin (10mg). Yet, there were 26 fewer deaths in the lower dose group. Unexpectedly, the total number of deaths from causes other than cardiac events was greater in the high dose group, exceeding those in the low dose group by 31. The lack of benefit was not loss on the New England Journal of Medicine who stated in their editorial that "further assurances as to the safety of this approach was needed" (NEJM 2005).

In 2011. H. Petursson *et al.*, examined cholesterol levels used in mortality risk algorithms in clinical guidelines based on ten years of prospective data from the Norwegian HUNT 2 study. The study population comprised 52,087 Norwegians, aged 20–74, who participated in the Nord-Trøndelag Health Study (HUNT 2)

tery disease, have demonstrated that statin drugs accelerate the progression of coronary artery calcification, as well, as abdominal aortic artery calcification. These results were confirmed by R. Nakazat *et al.*, in 2012, analyzing statins use and coronary artery plaque composition based on results from the International Multicenter CONFIRM Registry. The authors identified 6,673 individuals (2,413 on statin therapy and 4,260 not on statin therapy) with no known CAD, and with available statin use status. They studied the relationship between statin use and the presence and extent of specific plaque composition types, which was graded as non-calcified (NCP), mixed (MP), or calcified (CP) plaque. Compared to the individuals not taking statins, those taking statins had a <u>higher</u> prevalence of risk factors and obstructive CAD leading the authors to conclude that statin use is associated with an increased prevalence and extent of coronary plaques possessing calcium.

Despite the published findings questioning the benefit of cholesterol lowering drugs, several pharmaceutical companies set out to develop a new class of cholesterol lowering drugs called CEPT inhibitors. A CETP inhibitor blocks the cholesterylester transfer protein (CETP), and are designed to substantially increases HDL-cholesterol, and reverse cholesterol transport.

The results of the ILLUMINATE trial were published in *The New England Journal of Medicine* in 2007. The trial involved 15,067 patients (mean age 61 years) with coronary heart disease (CHD), or at risk for CHD (type

2 diabetes). Patients underwent a run-in period of 4-10 weeks during which they received lifestyle counseling, with or without atorvastatin (statin), to achieve a low-density lipoprotein cholesterol (LDL-C) goal of <100 mg/dl. Patients who achieved that target at the end of the run-in period were randomized to atorvastatin at the dose established during run-in, plus torcetrapib 60 mg (CETP inhibitor), or placebo. The trial was planned to run for 4.5 years.

At 12 months, patients who received torcetrapib showed an unprecedented panel of cholesterol results, including:

- Mean increase of 72.1% in HDL-cholesterol;
- Mean decrease of 24.9% in LDL-cholesterol; and
- Small mean decrease of 9% in triglycerides compared with baseline.

These lipid effects were consistent with those in previous studies.

The primary endpoint of the trial was a composite of first major cardiovascular event, defined as coronary heart disease (CHD) death, nonfatal myocardial infarction (MI), stroke, or hospitalization for unstable angina. At termination, the torcetrapib group showed a 25% increased risk over the groups that received atorvastatin alone.

If the deposition of cholesterol in the plaques is not due to LDL, then some altered form of lipoprotein must be responsible. It seems that only a fraction of the

LDL universe is atherogenic, with the majority of circulating LDL not contributing to coronary disease. Therefore, the reduction of total LDL-cholesterol as a target for hypolipidemic treatment for prevention of atherosclerosis is chasing after the wrong blood marker.

Particularly atherogenic forms of LDL include small, dense LDL particles and oxidized LDL. The small dense LDL particles are manufactured in the liver in response to fructose in the diet. Studies have shown that fructose (a sugar found in fruit) ingestion is associated with a decrease of LDL particle size and an increase in its density. This effect is not limited to fructose either, since sucrose (table sugar) breaks down to glucose and fructose when ingested. High-carbohydrate diets therefore reduce plasma LDL cholesterol, but also provokes the appearance of an atherogenic lipoprotein profile, characterized by high plasma triglycerides, small dense LDL particles, and reduced HDL cholesterol.

The pathogenesis of atherosclerosis begins with injury to the endothelial cells lining the medium and large arteries. The injury to the endothelial cells allows small LDL particles to enter into the intima leading to an accumulation of cholesterol in this space.

The knowledge that LDL-cholesterol is extremely susceptible to oxidative damage has been known for some time. To date, there are over 10,000 journal articles on oxidized LDL. It is now clear from the large volume of literature, that oxidized LDL cholesterol is a critical factor in the development of atherosclerosis.

Oxidized LDL (Ox-LDL) is chemotactic for monocytes (Chemotaxis is the movement of a cell in response to a chemical stimulus). In other words, monocytes are attracted to the Ox-LDL particle through scavenger receptors binding on the monocyte. Following binding to the ox-LDL particle, monocytes transform themselves into macrophages. Ox-LDL binds with high affinity to the scavenger receptors on the macrophage plasma membrane, which leads to the internalization of the Ox-LDL and lead to its degradation (Figure 17).

The macrophage engulfs the Ox-LDL particle eventually becoming a "Foam cell". The conversion of

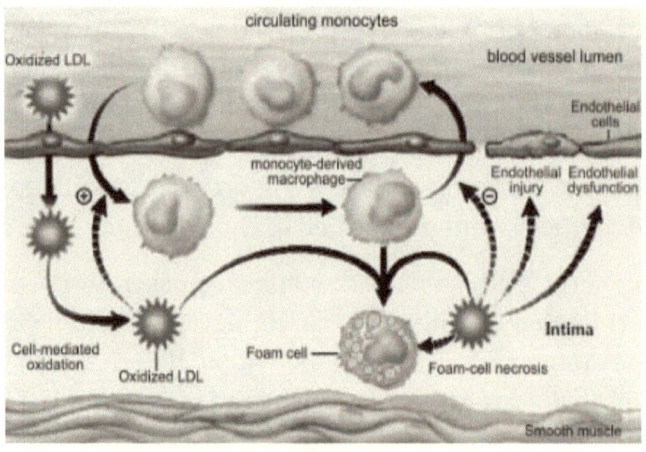

Figure 17: Oxidized cholesterol triggers the migration of monocyte/macrophage which engulf the LDL particle. The cholesterol engorged macrophage transform into foam cells which eventually die forming the plaque seen in atherosclerosis.

monocyte-to-macrophage differentiation is specific to Ox-LDL, and not native LDL. It is also dependent on the extent of LDL oxidation, and requires Ox-LDL internalization by the cells. The lipid-laden "foam cells" observed in early atherosclerotic lesions appear to be monocyte/macrophages that have taken up cholesterol in the intimal space. Malondialdehyde, from peroxidized polyunsaturated fatty acids, induces avid uptake of cholesterol by the scavenger receptor of human monocyte-macrophages!

The Polyunsaturated Fat Hypothesis

As mentioned previously, atherosclerosis begins with injury to the endothelial cells lining medium and large arteries. There is significant evidence that suggests exposure to dietary unsaturated fatty acids can directly affect endothelial cell metabolism. Significant amounts of data have been accumulated to show that linoleic acid can induce discernable injury to endothelial cells in blood vessels. An internet search using the search term "linoleic acid and endothelial dysfunction" will yield over 146,000 hits. Using the same parameters, but substituting arachidonic acid, will yield over 178,000 hits! This vast amount of data leads to one conclusion: these *n-6* fatty acids damage the endothelial walls of arteries.

The effects of n-6 fatty acids on endothelial cells are numerous. There is a significant increase in adhesion of monocytes to the endothelial monolayer in the presence of n-6 fatty acids. These unsaturated fats are involved in oxidative stress, cellular dysfunction, mitochondrial dysfunction, inflammation, and apoptosis (cell death). So, from this we can postulate that n-6 fatty acids can induce the first step in atherosclerosis – endothelial injury.

As endothelial cell undergo injury, they release endothelial microparticles (EMP) which can be measured as an index of endothelial injury and dysfunction. Microparticles are small vesicles that are released from cells through plasma membrane budding, leading to the formation of membrane blebs.

Acute endothelial injury, such as that induced by secondhand smoke, rapidly compromises endothelial function and increases circulating EMP in healthy subjects. Therefore, endothelial microparticles are a useful marker for endothelial injury.

Studies have shown that meals rich in *n-6* polyunsaturated vegetable oil, irrespective of whether it has been oxidized through heating, causes injury to the vascular endothelium, resulting in increased shedding of endothelial microparticles. **Healthy subjects given meals enriched with either unheated or heated sunflower oil have elevated levels of endothelial microparticles one hour after consuming the meal.** However, this phenomenon is not observed in individuals consuming saturated fats. The subjects who ate the polyunsaturated oil had a 20% increase in endothelial microparticles!

We know that atherosclerosis is not the result of the uptake of native LDL, which itself is incapable of causing cholesterol accumulation in monocyte/macrophages, but instead is due to the uptake of one or more modified forms of LDL. What is the source of this modified LDL? This is the subject of some debate. But it is clear that diet plays a significant role; especially with linoleic acid oxidation products.

If we look at the composition of the atherosclerotic plaque for clues, we find high levels of hydroxyoctadecanoic acids (derived from linoleic acid), 15-hydroxyeicosatetranoic acid (derived from arachidonic acid), and 11-HETE (derived from arachidonic acid) in all atherosclerotic plaques. Low levels of 9-oxo-octadecanoic acid (from linoleic acid), and 13-oxoODE from linoleic acid) are also present. What is important to note from these observations is the compounds found in the plaques are the oxidation products of linoleic and arachidonic acid, both polyunsaturated omega-6 fatty acids found in vegetable oils.

An article in the lancet in 1994 looked at dietary polyunsaturated fatty acids and composition of human aortic plaques. It compared the fatty acid composition of post-mortem blood samples to the fatty acids composition of aortic plaques and adipose tissue (adipose tissue, or body fat reflects the dietary intake of fatty acids). While there were no associations with saturated fatty acids, they did conclude that there is "a direct influence of dietary polyunsaturated fatty acids on aortic plaque formation and suggest that current trends favoring increased intake of polyunsaturated fatty acids should be reconsidered."

Another study examined 50 subjects with coronary artery disease (>50% stenosis in one or more major coronary vessels), and 54 without coronary artery disease, looking at systemic levels of specific fatty acid oxidation products. They found 9-HETE and F(2)-isoprostanes, were significantly elevated in patients with coronary artery disease. Both are oxidation products of arachidonic acid, again supporting the hypothesis that *n-6* polyunsaturated fatty acids are responsible for plaque formation in coronary artery disease.

Studies going back to 1997 show that the oxidation products in atherosclerotic plaques are oxidation products of linoleic and arachidonic acid, both polyunsaturated fats. Gniwotta *et al.*, in 1997 concluded the "data show that human atherosclerotic lesions contain increased amounts of hydroxyl-linoleic acid isomers and isoprostanes when compared with non-atherosclerotic vessel wall and suggest a link between local lipid peroxidation and progression of atherosclerosis."

Waddington *et al.*, in 2003, published an article describing the presence of fatty acid oxidation products in histological samples of atherosclerosis plaque. They found, as have others, that arachidonic acid oxidation products were significantly higher in those subjects who also had coronary artery disease.

From this evidence, one can deduce that linoleic acid is a precursor to the oxidized linoleic metabolites found in atherosclerotic plaques. Humans cannot synthesize linoleic acid, so our diet is the sole source of linoleic acid in humans. These linoleic acid stores, in turn, serve as the source of endogenous oxidized linoleic metabolites, although oxidized linoleic metabolites are obtained via the diet as well. Studies have shown that lowering dietary linoleic acid from 6.7% to 2.4% of calories can significantly lower oxidized linoleic metabolites.

Studies have also demonstrated that oxidized polyunsaturated fatty acid products, including oxidized linoleic acid, are absorbed by the small intestine and incorporated into chylomicrons. Increased peroxide levels are seen in chylomicrons, VLDL, and LDL lipoproteins. Therefore, oxidized linoleic acid products are efficiently incorporated into the LDL particle leading to ox-LDL. The oxidation of lipoproteins does not just result in the creation of a single molecular species, but a variety of oxidation products. One specific target of LDL oxidation that is of particular importance is the Apo B lipoprotein on the LDL particle. As LDL-particle undergoes oxidation, the products of lipid peroxidation (such as HNE or other aldehyde products derived from lipid peroxidation), bind to the lysine residues on Apo B. This results in the modification of the Apo B molecule which induces a recognition by the scavenger receptor on tissue macrophages.

So, what does all of this mean? When rabbits are fed a diet rich in oxidized lipid, there is a 100% increase in fatty streak lesions in the aorta and a >100% increase in total cholesterol in the pulmonary artery. Additionally, when rats are fed oxidized corn oil, there is a significantly increased aortic wall thickness after just six months of dietary feeding.

Epidemiological evidence

If LDL-cholesterol levels were the cause of atherosclerosis, then we would expect the incidence of coronary artery disease to be similar across different geographies and populations. However, this is not the case.

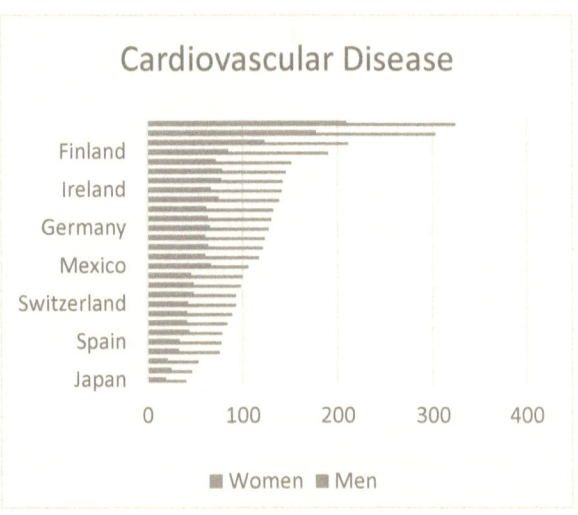

Figure 18: Incidence of cardiovascular disease age-standardized rates per 100,000 of the population.

As you can see in Figure 18, the incidence of cardiovascular disease in the United States is significantly higher than other countries, suggesting that dietary factors are in play.

The age adjusted incidence of cardiovascular disease in the United State is 145 cases per 100,000 people. Compare this rate to Japan, France, or Korea whose rates are 66% lower than the US rate for cardiovascular disease, and you must conclude that some other factor is in play. One obvious difference is diet.

A dietary aspect we should be able to dismiss is the hypothesis that consumption of saturated fat is somehow correlated to cardiovascular disease. Despite

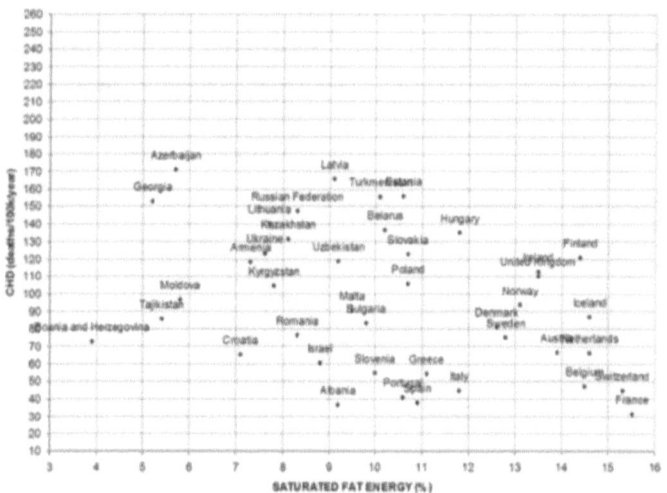

Figure 19: Percent of saturated fat energy (%) vs Coronary Heart disease deaths/100,000/year) in European men 1998.

recommendations to reduce the amount of saturated fat in the diet, there is no correlation between saturated fat and deaths due to coronary heart disease when comparing different geographies, as shown in Figure 19. In fact, France has the highest consumption of saturated fat and the lowest rate of heart disease! Given what we have discussed previously on saturated fat, it does not appear saturated fats have an impact on deaths due to coronary heart disease.

However, if we look at arachidonic acid content of adipose tissue in across different countries, and compare this to heart disease mortality, we see a different picture, and a clear correlation with arachidonic acid (20:4 polyunsaturated fat) and cardiac mortality (Figure 20).

Let's next look at populations that have not been exposed to seed oils, which are few. A study published in the journal of *Tropical and Geographical Medicine* found that coronary heart disease is virtually unknown in the

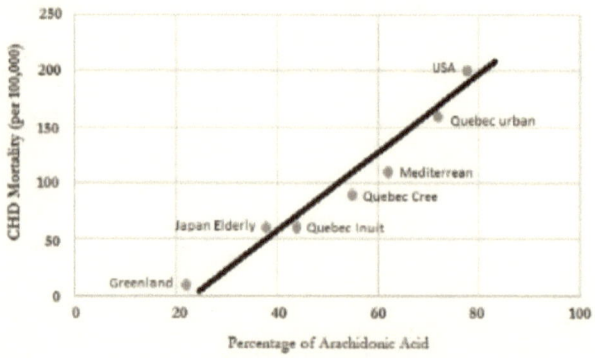

Figure 20: Mortality rates due to heart disease and tissue arachidonic acid.

Vedda population of Sri Lanka. The Vedda communities in the South-Eastern jungles of Sri Lanka consume a diet of fruits, yams, coconuts, and hunting wild game. The majority of dietary fat in the traditional Vedda population comes from coconut and wild game, both high in saturated fat.

The study examined 207 adults between 20-83 years of age. A detailed medical history was taken of each subject, which included level of daily physical activity, dietary and smoking habits. A complete physical examination and blood analysis was performed with special attention to cardiovascular diseases.

None of the subjects reported heart related problems despite the fact that 39% of the men smoked, and only 3.8% had elevated blood pressure. Electrocardiograms showed no evidence of heart disease.

Even with the high saturated fat diet, total cholesterol as well as triglyceride levels were comparable those of the Sri Lanka population. The chief difference is they consume little polyunsaturated fats and no vegetable oils.

In 1978, Sri Lanka had a very low rate of coronary heart disease as well, representing one (1) death per 100,000 of the population. As with most countries though, the importation of polyunsaturated vegetable oils increased over time and consequently, the use of coconut oil decreased as the result of a cheaper alternative to traditional coconut oil. According to WHO statistics from 2012, ischemic heart disease was (and still is) the leading cause of death in Sri Lanka, killing 32,6000 people per year. Today, Sri Lanka has a death rate from ischemic heart disease of 66 deaths per 100,000 which is in line with the countries in the lower end of the cardiovascular disease rate in Figure 18. This is lower than the western countries, but still, this represents a 66% increase from 1978!

There are other populations with little cardio-vascular disease and no vegetable oil consumption, despite their relatively high saturated fat diet. The Pukapuka and Tokalau populations live on atolls in the northern Cook island. These Polynesians eat a diet that consists mainly of breadfruit, fish and coconuts, although pork and chickens are consumed occasionally. Flour, sugar and canned meats arrive by boat every couple of months. The diet is low on unsaturated fats and no vegetable oils.

The consumption of coconut is higher in the Tokalau (63%) than the Pukapuka (36%). Therefore, the amount of saturated fat is higher in the Tokalau, and is reflected by an increase of 35-40mg/dl of total cholesterol over the Pukapuka.

Biopsies from adipose tissue show both groups have 10-12% lauric acid (12:0 saturated fat), and 16-17% myristic acid (14:0 saturated fat). Total groups have tissue saturated fats of 52-53% while unsaturated fats constitute 47-48% of adipose fat. The unsaturated fats are mostly monounsaturated fats. This is compared to adipose tissue samples in New Zealand Europeans containing 34% saturated fat and 64% unsaturated fats.

Despite the high saturated fat diet, coronary heart disease is essentially non-existent. And there is no evidence that the high saturated fat diet has a harmful effect on either population, but strongly suggests the absence of vegetable oils in the diet may be responsible for the low incidence of cardiovascular disease.

In summary, we know that vegetable oils are deteriorated by repeated heating that leads to lipid peroxidation. The omega-6 polyunsaturated fats and their metabolites cause vascular inflammation, as well as vascular changes, which predispose oneself to atherosclerosis. This vascular inflammation appears to be the triggering episode, leading to the cascading events that result in atherosclerosis. Continued consumption of omega-6 polyunsaturated fats and their metabolites leads to oxy-LDL formation and modification of the Apo B protein. This causes a recognition by tissue monocytes which engulf the LDL-particle and become trapped, leading ultimately to the deposits of cholesterol in the intima of the coronary arteries (and elsewhere). And this is repeated with every meal where polyunsaturated (and monounsaturated) fats are consumed, again due to the reactivity of the double bonds in unsaturated fats.

The inflammatory aspect of atherosclerosis is extremely important to the pathology of the disease. We will explore the role of vegetable oils and their impact on inflammation in subsequent chapters. As we explore other organ systems, you will begin to see the interrelationship of other inflammatory conditions and cardiovascular disease, all leading back to vegetable oils.

5. Polyunsaturated Fats and Cancer

I have long believed that cancer is a mitochondrial disease. Indeed, there are many characteristics of cancer that suggest that cancer either results from, or is exacerbated, by mitochondrial dysfunction. I suggest this dysfunction is the result of changes in mitochondrial structure caused by the direct incorporation of peroxidized unsaturated fatty acids into the mitochondrial membrane, by affecting the apoptotic pathway in the mitochondria, and by the formation of DNA adducts as a consequence of peroxized fatty acids. In addition, polyunsaturated oils, which are rich is n-6 fatty acids can contribute to cancer development through the inflammatory process.

In 1926, Otto Warburg found that cancer cells preferentially used glycolysis for ATP production, and that there is a correlation between the degree of conversion to glycolysis and the aggressiveness of the tumor cells. Warburg assumed that such 'aerobic glycolysis' was a universal property of malignant cells and suggested that cancer is caused by impaired mitochondrial metabolism. Quoting Warburg, *"...all normal body cells are thus obligate aerobes, whereas all cancer cells are partial anaerobes. From the standpoint of the physics and chemistry of life this difference between normal and cancer cells is so great that one can scarcely picture a greater difference. Oxygen gas, the donor of energy in plants and animals is dethroned in the cancer cells and replaced by an energy yielding reaction of the lowest living forms, namely, a fermentation of glucose."* Warburg showed that cells could be transformed into cancerous ones by subjecting them to periods of low oxygen exposure. Moreover, he showed that once cells had converted to a cancerous state, the process was not reversible.

Mitochondrial dysregulation is one of the most common hallmarks of cancer, and we are witnessing a renaissance of Warburg's fundamental observation. Studies during the past decade have shed light on some of the peculiarities of mitochondrial function in cancer cells. There are seven known essential alterations in cells that characterize malignant change: 1) self-sufficiency in the ability to divide and grow without growth signals, 2) an overall insensitivity to factors that inhibit growth, 3) a sustained and unlimited ability to divide (immortal cells), 4) creation of new blood vessels form from pre-existing vessels (angiogenesis), 5) tissue invasion and metastasis, 6) evasion of programmed cell death (apoptosis), and 7) the preferential use of the glycolytic pathway.

Unfortunately, a significant amount of capital and research has been diverted into genetic changes as the ultimate cause of cancer. But despite 90 years of intensive research focused on a genetic cause, no single cause for cancer has been established. We have known since 1970's that the nucleus is not the driver of cancer development. However, the prevailing hypothesis continues to be that cancer arises as a result of genetic mutations.

While many oncogenes and tumor suppressor genes have been identified, we also know that the nucleus can be "reprogrammed" into a normal cell. In 1975, Mintz and Illmensee took malignant mouse teratocarcinoma cells and demonstrated that teratocarcinoma cells when inserted into a germ line, will ultimately give rise to adult mice. The authors concluded that *"the results also furnish an unequivocal example in animals of a non-mutational basis for transformation to malignancy and of reversal to normalcy. "*In a frog renal carcinoma model, the transfer of nuclei from tumor cells into oocytes was reported to reverse oncogenesis and to direct development to the tadpole stage. In 2003, Li, *et al.*

concluded that "tumor cells can be epigenetically repro-grammed into normal cell types". They based this ob-servation on experiments where they took medulloblas-toma nuclei and cloned them to form normal mouse em-bryos.

There are several things in common with all of the nuclear transfer experiments. The uncontrolled pro-liferation is suppressed and normal patterns of differen-tiation are restored. The cancer cells were repro-grammed when inserted into the oocyte. It is possible that there exists some yet unknown signaling mecha-nism to transform the malignant DNA within the oo-cyte. However, we do know the nucleus in these exper-iments was removed from its environment with dys-functional mitochondria, into an oocyte with normal mi-tochondria!

Let look at those elements of commonality in cancer cells. Warburg proposed that cancer cells prefer-entially used glycolysis for ATP (energy) production, and that there is a correlation between the degree of con-version to glycolysis and the aggressiveness of the tu-mor cells. Glycolysis (from glycose, an older term for glucose + -lysis degradation) is the metabolic pathway that converts glucose (sugar), into pyruvate. Glycolysis is an anaerobic (or oxygen independent) metabolic path-way, meaning that it does not use molecular oxygen for any of its reactions. These reactions take place in the cy-toplasm of the cell. In a normal cell, pyruvate is trans-ported into the mitochondria to undergo aerobic (using oxygen) metabolism via the Krebs citric acid cycle. Rapidly growing tumor cells typically have glycolytic rates that are up to 200 times higher than those of their normal tissues of origin!

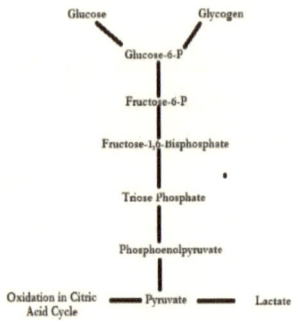

Figure 21: Glycolysis. Glucose is ultimately converted to pyruvate. Normally pyruvate is further metabolized in the citric acid (Krebs) cycle. In cancer, pyruvate is converted into lactic acid.

Glycolysis is one of the most ancient metabolic pathways and occurs, with variations, in nearly all organisms. Davila and Zamorano hypothesized in 2013 that cancer represent a regression to the earliest stage of evolution. This reversion is triggered by the dysregulation of the mitochondria due to cumulative oxidative damage to mitochondrial and nuclear DNA. As a result, the normal, differentiated cell gradually reverts to the phenotype of a facultative anaerobic, optimized for survival and proliferation in hypoxic environments (a facultative anaerobe is an organism that can use oxygen but also has anaerobic methods of energy production. It can survive in either environment).

Aerobic respiration, as seen in Figure 22, converts pyruvate and ultimately breaks it down to carbon

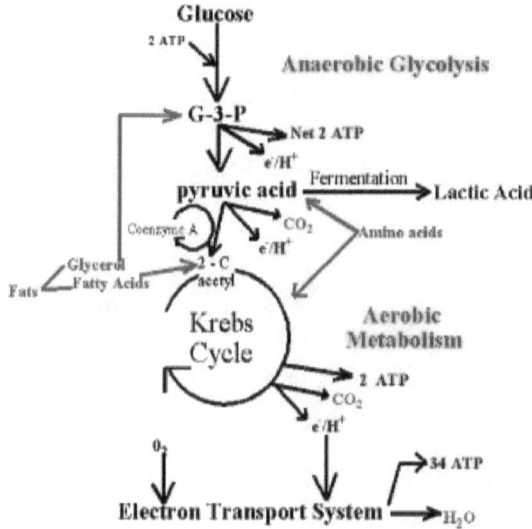

Figure 22: Aerobic Respiration. Pyruvate enters the Citric Acid (or Krebs) cycle ultimately breaking down into carbon dioxide and water.

dioxide (CO_2) and water (H_2O). It consists of two parts: the Krebs cycle and the electron transport system. Aerobic respiration is considered the evolutionary newer pathway. Where four (4) ATP molecules are created during glycolysis, thirty-six (36) ATP molecules are formed during aerobic metabolism. It is no wonder that the cancer cell requires so much glucose!

The Mitochondria

Mitochondria are present in both plant and animal cells. They are rod-shaped structures that are enclosed within two membranes (Figure 23). The outer membrane is completely permeable to nutrient molecules. The inner membrane is more complex in structure than the outer membrane and contains the complexes of the electron transport chain. It is permeable only to oxygen, carbon dioxide and water. The inner membrane has folding called the cristae that increase the surface area. The Krebs cycle and electron transport system take place within the walls of the mitochondria.

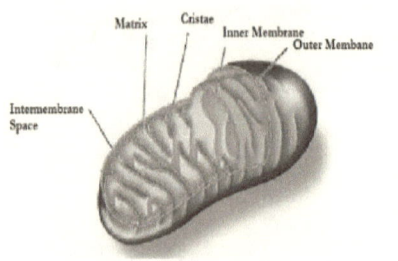

Figure 23: The mitochondria. The Krebs cycle and electron transport system take place within the walls of the mitochondria.

The inner mitochondrial membrane can be regarded as a complex lipoprotein structure due to the strong functional interactions between its constituent proteins and <u>phospholipids.</u>

Phospholipids are a class of lipids that are a major component of all cell membranes. Of the three major phospholipids that comprise the mitochondrial walls, <u>cardiolipin</u>, although having the lowest abundance (approximately 20%), is highly specific to the inner mitochondrial membrane

Cardiolipin is both a major structural and functional phospholipid of mitochondria. It is responsible for a wide range of mitochondrial functions, and is found on all membranes that synthesize ATP. This ubiquitous, and intimate association between cardiolipin and energy forming membranes indicates an important role for cardiolipin in mitochondrial energy production. Therefore, changes in the structure of cardiolipin can cause many pathological conditions, including the potential of causing the mitochondrial dysfunction we see in cancer. Cardiolipin in mammalian mitochondria typically have 4 polyunsaturated linoleic acid chains which are subject to oxidation. This oxidation leads to "reactive oxygen species" we discussed previously

There are several ways in which unsaturated fats can disrupt mitochondrial function. First, the overall lipid content of the cardiolipin molecule can be altered. As mentioned previously, cardiolipin consists of four polyunsaturated linoleic acid chains. Because of the ubiquitous nature of the cardiolipin molecule, the content of the fatty acids are well preserved across species and is commonly viewed as highly regulated due to its high levels of linoleic acid (18:2, $n-6$). However, the lipid structure of cardiolipin is dependent on dietary fats. For instance, when linoleic and docosahexaenoic acid (22:6, $n-3$) are present in the same diet, docosahexaenoic acid is incorporated into cardiolipin at the expense of linoleic acid. In fact, Cardiolipin is very diet-responsive. Cardiolipin has been modified experimentally to contain 85–90% linoleic acid (18:2 $n-6$), 50% docosahexaenoic acid (DHA, 22:6 $n-3$), or 50% oleic acid (18:1 $n-9$) by changing the fatty acid composition of the diet. There is a strong correlation between the degree of cardiolipin fatty acid unsaturation, and mitochondrial efficiency. Indeed, research suggests that any disturbance of the CL profile may result in mitochondrial dysfunction. This has been well documented in a variety of diseases associated with mitochondrial dysfunction.

Sapandowski, *et al.*, have shown that Cardiolipin composition is easily modified in prostate cancer cells. The authors took tumor cells from prostate cancer patients and exposed them to different fatty acids in cell culture. The composition of mitochondrial cardiolipin was easily modified by the fatty acids in the culture media. Cardiolipin had a higher concentration of palmitoleic acid in five out of six patients, compared to normal prostate tissue (palmitoleic acid is a *n-7* monosaturated fatty acid).

In addition, there is evidence to suggest that the mitochondrial dysfunction seen in cancer cells may reflect a problem of cardiolipin synthesis. Kiebish *et al.* observed major abnormalities in cardiolipin content or composition in different mouse brain tumors (astrocytoma, ependymoblastoma, and micro-glioma). The abnormalities in cardiolipin include an abundance of immature forms of the molecule, and deficiencies in the mature form suggesting major defects in cardiolipin synthesis and remodeling. They noted the tumor cardiolipin abnormalities were also associated with significant reductions in function of the electron transport chain supporting the original observations of Warburg.

In 1927, Bernstein and Elias published *Lipoids and Carcinoma Growth* where they reported that diets that are low in unsaturated fatty acids prevented the development of spontaneous tumors. Subsequent researchers have concluded that unsaturated fats are essential for the growth of tumors. By 1981, it was generally accepted that *n*-6 polyunsaturated fatty acids have tumor-promoting activity in experimental models. Karmali *et al.* first reported a difference in the effects of *n*-3 and *n*-6 polyunsaturated fatty acids on the growth of transplantable mammary tumors. The group observed the tumor-promoting activity of *n*-6 polyunsaturated fatty acids was abrogated by competitive inhibition by *n*-3 polyunsaturated fatty.

Several studies have shown that diets containing corn oil, with its high levels of *n*-6 PUFAs (such as linoleic acid), enhances breast and colon tumorigenesis in rodents, whereas fish oil, reduces carcinogenesis. When rats were fed diets containing different levels of linoleic acid, mammary tumorigenesis increased proportionately in the range of 0.5 to 4.4% of dietary linoleate, showing tumorigenesis is very sensitive to linoleic acid in the diet.

Fay *et al.* conducted a meta-analysis extracted from 97 studies involving 12,800 mice and rats looking at the effect of saturated, monounsaturated and polyunsaturated fats on the incidence of mammary tumors. The results show that *n*-6 polyunsaturated fats have a strong correlation while saturated fats have a weak tumor enhancing effect; *n*-3 polyunsaturated fats had a weak protective effect and monounsaturated fats had no effect. Of interesting note is the effect was greater when the *n*-

6 polyunsaturated fat intake was >4% to the total caloric intake!

Having more omega-3 fatty acids is not the answer either. Song *et al.* noted that polyunsaturated (*n*-3) fatty acids, are increased in plasma and tissue lipids of rats fed docosahexaenoic acid-containing (DHA) oils. In other words, incorporation of high amounts of (n-3) fatty acids (mainly DHA from fish oils) can disrupt cardiolipin because of the susceptibility of membranes to lipid peroxidation. In addition, high amounts of polyunsaturated oil can overwhelm the antioxidant system leading to more peroxidation of mitochondrial structures.

Background studies of dietary omega-3 fatty acid intake and prostate cancer risk are inconsistent. Several studies have shown that omega-3 fatty acids reduce prostate tumor growth, slowed histopathological progression, and increased survival, whereas omega-6 fatty acids had opposite effects.

However, recent large prospective studies have found an increase in the risk of prostate cancer among men with high blood concentrations of long-chain omega-3 polyunsaturated fatty acids, the type found in fish oils. The Selenium and Vitamin E Cancer Prevention Trial studied 834 men diagnosed with prostate cancer, of which 156 had high-grade cancer. They found an association between omega-3 fatty acids and prostate cancer risk overall as well as by cancer grade. They concluded, as with other reports, of an increased prostate cancer risk among men with high blood concentrations of omega-3 fats, and suggested that these fatty acids are involved in prostate tumorigenesis.

Similar results were found in the Prostate Cancer Prevention Trial. In a study involving 1,658 prostate cancer patients, docosahexaenoic acid was positively associated with high-grade disease. The study findings are contrary to those expected from the anti-inflammatory effects of this omega-3 fatty acid.

The European Prospective Investigation into Cancer and Nutrition found a similar relationship between omega-3 fatty acids and high-risk prostate cancer. The study was an analysis of 962 men with a diagnosis of prostate cancer and 1061 matched controls. They reported significant positive associations between alpha-linolenic, and eicosapentaenoic acids (omega-3 fatty acids) and risk of high-grade prostate cancer.

A study at the Fred Hutchinson Cancer Research Center looked at high-heat cooking methods and an increase in the risk of prostate cancer. They examined the association between the intake of deep-fried foods from a food frequency questionnaire (French fries, fried chicken, fried fish, doughnuts and snack chips) and prostate cancer risk. They found that regular consumption of select deep-fried foods is associated with increased prostate cancer. In fact, consuming more than one (1) portion of these deep-fried foods per week increased prostate cancer risk between 27% and 35%! Additionally, there appears to be a trend toward more aggressive prostate cancer compared with less aggressive

prostate cancer, with increased risk of aggressive prostate cancer ranging between 38% and 41% for the highest compared with the lowest intake of these deep-fried
foods.

The Agency for Healthcare Research and Quality (AHRQ), through its Evidence-Based Practice Centers (EPCs), sponsored the development of evidence reports *Effects of Omega-3 Fatty Acids on Cancer*. The EPC
screened 4,834 titles, reviewed 356 articles, and included
52 articles in their review of the tumor incidence and
outcomes after cancer treatment. They found only six
were statistically significant. Significant associations between omega-3 consumption (in the form of both fish
and alpha-linolenic acid) and cancer risk were reported
for breast cancer in two studies; for lung cancer in two;
for prostate cancer in one; and for skin cancer in one. For
breast cancer one significant estimate was for increased
risk and one was for decreased risk; five other estimates
did not show a significant association. For lung cancer
one of the significant associations was for increased cancer risk, the other was for decreased risk and four other
estimates were not significant.

They concluded that in a large body of literature
spanning numerous cohorts from many countries with
different demographic characteristics, does not suggest
a significant association between omega-3 fatty acids
and cancer incidence. One can explain the variance in
outcome is due to the instability of omega-3 fatty acids
being prone to oxidation. Unless the omega-3 fatty acids

are under constant refrigeration and not exposed to oxygen, they are readily oxidized.

Work from Sasaki *et al.* support concern over the use of omega-3 fatty acids to reduce tumor formation. They observed that an increase in the n-3/n-6 ratio did not suppress the incidence or reduce the latency of mammary tumor development. Instead, as the n-3/n-6 ratios were elevated, the total number and weight of tumors increased gradually!

Apoptosis

Apoptosis is the process of programmed death. It is a highly regulated pathway that occurs in all multicellular organisms. Between 50 and 70 billion cells die each day due to apoptosis in the average human adult. Apoptosis is the most common physiological form of cell death and occurs during embryonic development, tissue modelling, immune regulation and tumor regression. In other words, tissues are always in a state of balance between proliferation and apoptosis. When apoptosis is inhibited, the result is uncontrolled proliferation of cells as seen in cancer.

It shouldn't come as a surprise that the process of apoptosis involves the mitochondria and fatty acids. Saturated fatty acids promote apoptosis while polyunsaturated fats inhibit the process. Saturated fatty acids induce apoptosis via multiple pathways (Figure 24).

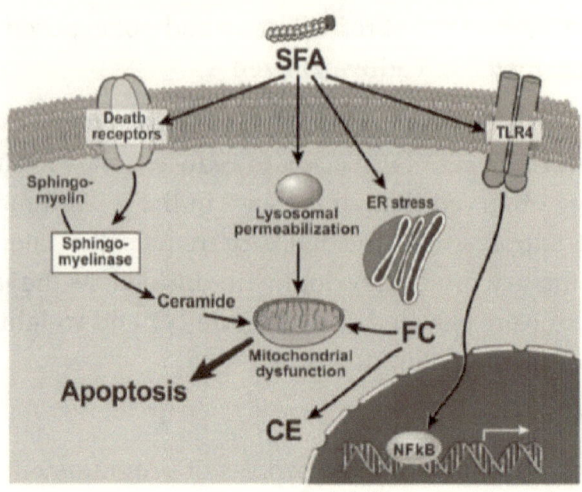

Figure 24: The mechanism of apoptosis.

There are a group of membrane receptors collectively called death receptors due to their ability to trigger the cell death. Tumor Necrosis Factor (TNF) was isolated more than 15 years ago, based on its ability to cause cell death, but did not fulfill initial expectations in the treatment of cancer due to its high toxicity. The TNF receptor is a death receptor found on all cells with the exception of red blood cells.

Saturated fatty acids bind to the death receptors embedded in the cell membrane. This receptor-SFA complex stimulates the production of ceramide which in turn initiates the cascade of changes in the mitochondria leading to cell death. Once the cell has undergone cell death, the remains are consumed by macrophages.

However, as typical in biology, there are alternative pathways to induce apoptosis. For example, saturated fatty acids induce "endoplasmic reticulum stress" and apoptosis independently of ceramide and the death receptor. Saturated fatty acids can directly induce mitochondrial dysfunction and oxidative stress through a process of lysosomal disruption. The take home message is the difference in fatty acid can direct whether a cell will undergo apoptosis by multiple pathways via the mitochondria.

One of the hallmarks of cancer is the failure of the cell to undergo apoptosis, and instead becomes immortal. It is now becoming clear that oncogenic mutations result in a disruption of the apoptosis process leading to tumor initiation, proliferation or metastasis. There are many cancer-related gene mutations that affect apoptosis. We are in the process of discovering that most cytotoxic cancer treatments induce apoptosis leading to the theory that treatment failure may be the result of mitochondrial dysfunction.

Hardy *et al.* report that unsaturated FFAs stimulated the proliferation of human breast cancer cells, whereas saturated FFAs inhibited it and caused apoptosis. Palmitate (a saturated fatty acid) decreased the mitochondrial membrane potential and caused cytochrome c release. Fauser *et al.* was able to induce apoptosis by lauric acid (a medium chain saturated fatty acid) in colon cancer cells due to induction of oxidative stress.

Berquin *et al.* found that omega-3 fatty acids reduced prostate tumor growth, slowed histopathological progression, and increased survival, in mice fed diets rich in either n-3 or n-6 fatty acids. Omega-6 fatty acids had opposite effects. These effects appeared to be related to the apoptotic pathway.

Oxidized Unsaturated Fatty Acids can Induce Changes

It has been proposed that the effect of dietary fat on cancer is the result of the activation of carcinogens by fat oxidation; products such as lipid hydroperoxides. In addition, peroxidized lipids can insert themselves into cellular membranes, and overwhelm cellular antioxidants. Thirdly, lipid peroxidation products can have a direct interaction on DNA.

As mentioned previously, Malondialdehyde is a naturally occurring product of lipid peroxidation. It is known to be both mutagenic and carcinogenic. Malondialdehyde reacts with DNA to form DNA adducts (a **DNA adduct** is when a piece of DNA is bonded to a cancer-causing chemical). In this case, Malondialdehyde forms a chemical bond to nuclear DNA.

Wang *et al.* analyzed DNA adducts induced by malondialdehyde, in surgical specimens of normal breast tissues of 51 breast cancer patients. Ten of the 51 cancer patients and 1 of the 28 controls were found to contain MDA adducts at the level of $> 1/10^{(7)}$ nucleotides. The authors concluded that the findings provide evidence that lipid peroxidation products can accumulate in human breast tissues and reach relatively high levels in the breast tissues of women with breast cancer.

There seems to be an interaction between these endogenous DNA modifications and carcinogen exposure-induced DNA adducts. Peluso *et al.*, tested breast fine-needle aspirate samples of 22 patients with breast cancer, at different clinical stages, compared to 13 controls. The results show that M_1dG adduct was higher in cancer cases than in controls and increased M_1dG was observed in women with a tumor grade 3.

Chole *et al.*, measured serum malondialdehyde level in 30 normal individuals and 30 patients each with confirmed oral precancerous, and oral cancer by pathology sections. The average serum malondialdehyde level in the control group was found to be 5.1 ηmol/ml. It was 9.3 ηmol/ml and 14.3 ηmol/ml in oral precancer and oral cancer, respectively. This is 2x and 3x the levels seen in controls. Therefore, malondialdehyde level was significant increase in serum malondialdehyde levels in the oral precancerous and oral cancer patients. Significant malondialdehyde levels have been seen in breast and lung cancer patients as well.

There is accumulating data that adducts from 4-HNE (another peroxidized fatty acid) are involved in the initiation and progression of cancer. 4-HNE can modulate a number of signaling processes mainly through forming adducts with proteins, nucleic acids, and membrane lipids. The formation of 4-HNE protein adducts in renal and colon cancer tissues has been related to the growth and progression of kidney and colon cancer. Increased levels of 4-HNE have been shown to be associated with liver cancer initiation in animal models and humans. 4-HNE may also contribute to cancer promotion by inhibiting DNA repair or by promoting inflammation.

In a study published in The Lancet in 1971, 846 men were assigned randomly to a conventional diet or to one similar in all respects except for a substitution of vegetable oils for saturated fat. At the end of the eight-year trial period, there was a greater incidence of fatal carcinomas in the experimental group. 31 of 174 deaths in the experimental group were due to cancer, as opposed to 17 of 178 deaths in the control group (P=0·06).

Epidemiological evidence

Lung cancer has been the leading cause of cancer death among women in Taiwan, Republic of China, since 1986. Cigarette smoking cannot fully explain the epidemiologic characteristics of lung cancer, especially with the increases seen in non-smokers. Taiwan is a country with significant wok cooking involving frying ingredients in vegetable oil exposing the cook to oil fumes. Studies in non-smokers have concluded that lung cancer risk is increased proportional to the number of meals per day. For women who cooked every day, the increase was threefold! The risk was also greater if women usually waited until fumes were emitted from the cooking oil before they began cooking. Lung cancer rates are higher in kitchen workers as well.

If we were to compare the consumption of polyunsaturated fatty acids in the US, we see a startling

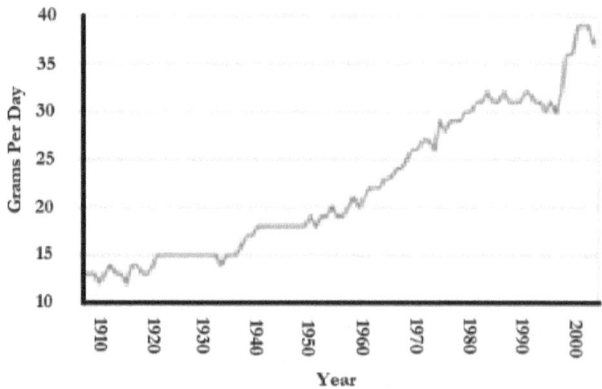

Figure 25: Polyunsaturated fatty acid consumption 1909 to 2005.

parallel. As the use of PUFA's increases, so do the lung cancer rates (Figure 25).

Lung cancer rates continue to rise despite all attempts to reduce tobacco consumption in the US. At a time that tobacco use is in decline, the incidence in lung cancers is increasing exponentially! In 1930, 80% of men smoked cigarettes and the tar content of cigarettes was much higher than it is today. The death rate at that time from lung cancer was very low. However, with the increase in consumption of PUFAs, lung cancer deaths have increased dramatically. By 1990, the number of American men who smoked had dropped to just 30%, but there were 60 times as many lung cancer deaths (Figure 26)!

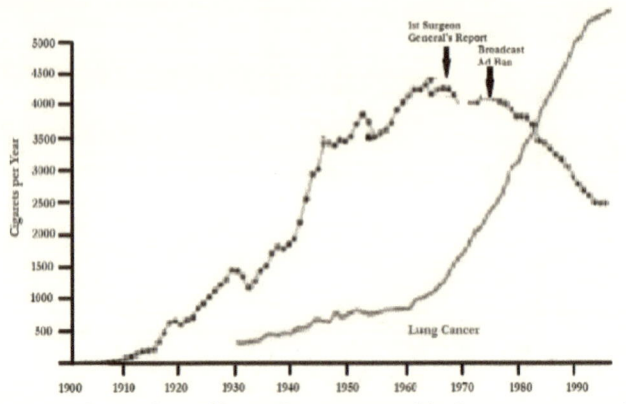

Figure 26: Comparison of Lung Cancer rates with cigarette consumption.

And the same holds true for prostate and other cancers. The rate for Prostate cancer has nearly tripled in 35 years (Figure 27).

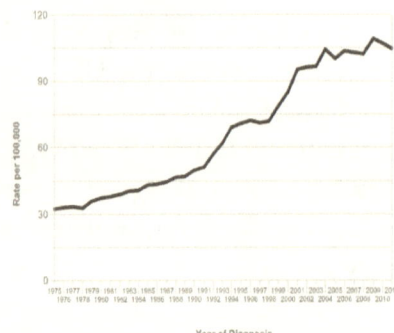

Figure 27: Prostate cancer incidence per 100,000 men from 1975 to 2010.

There is significant disparity among countries in term of cancer incidence. This suggests that while there may be a background rate, something is greatly affecting these population. One of the obvious variables is introduction of the western diet (vegetable oils). But there are many other environmental factors which compounds the issue.

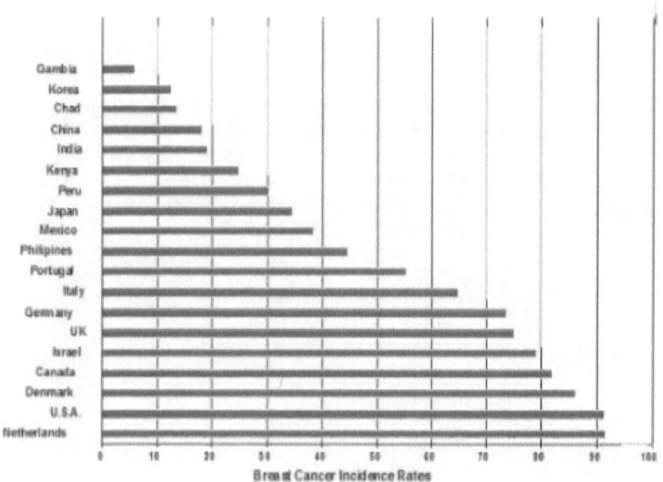

Figure 28: Breast Cancer Incidence per 100,000.

Since cancer develops at a slow rate over the course of many years, there aren't any prospective clinical trials to validate the hypothesis. In the absence of clinical data, we turn to correlations. If we look at polyunsaturated fatty acid consumption by region, a signal begins to appear. Those countries with higher PUFA consumption have higher rates of cancer. Take the Israeli paradox for example, where Israelis eat a diet which is approximately 30 grams a day. "The percentage of linoleic acid in the adipose tissue of the average Israelis is 24% as compared to 16% in Americans and less than 10% in many northern Europeans". The incidence of breast cancer in Israel is among the highest in the world. It is estimated that one in every eight Israeli women are at risk of developing breast cancer. In addition, they have the world's highest rate of non-Hodgkin's lymphoma.

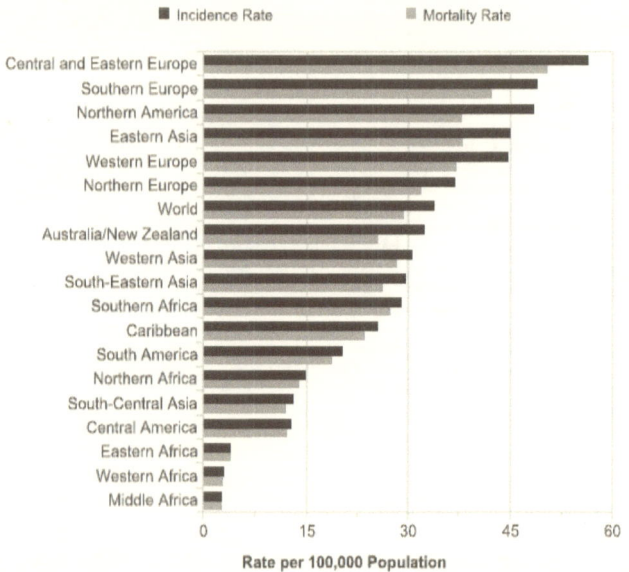

Figure 29: World Wide Lung Cancer Rates per 100,000 population.

Immunology

It has been well established that inflammation is a precursor to cancer formation. And the current area of promising cancer therapy treatment is immunotherapy. The premise is the immune system keeps cancer in check until it is overwhelmed or the cancer somehow "cloaks" itself from the immune system. The idea is everyone has cancer, but it is not manifested because the immune system destroys those cancerous cells before they form tumors. Therefore, a weakened immune system may determine whether a cancer progresses or not.

One significant piece of information to support the premise that the immune system affects the outcome of cancer, is the use of aspirin. Aspirin suppressed the production of prostaglandins and thromboxanes which are involved with inflammation. The study that elucidates aspirin's anticancer effects is the large meta-analysis of eight clinical studies involving regular aspirin use, which was published on January 1, 2011, in *The Lancet*. The analysis showed a substantial reduction in mortality for a number of different cancers. The importance of this is information is the fact the polyunsaturated fatty acids are closely tied to the immune system. Inflammation can be exacerbated with intake of *n-6* polyunsaturated fatty acids as well as being immunosuppressive. Since polyunsaturated fatty acids are directly associated with inflammatory-based pathology in such diseases as cancer, rheumatoid arthritis, atherosclerosis, and obesity, we will explore this association in depth in the next chapter.

6. Immune Suppression and Inflammation

A review of the previous chapters makes for a very strong argument that immune dysfunction may be causally related to tumorigenesis, as well as cardiovascular disease, and that the interrelationships are due to dietary fats. Current research indicates that diets high in n-6 unsaturated fat have been shown to be good promoters of tumorigenesis, as well as cardiovascular disease, and are also immunosuppressive relative to diets that are high in saturated fatty acids.

In the early days of organ transplantation, there

was a need for immunosuppressive drugs to stop transplant rejection. There was anecdotal evidence that since sunflower seeds were useful in treating autoimmune diseases, sunflower oil could be used prevent kidney transplants rejection. Studies have shown that diets high in polyunsaturated fat result in the inability to reject skin allografts.

To prove the point, a double-blind controlled study was undertaken to assess polyunsaturated fatty acids in human transplantation. Eighty-nine (89) patients were studied and followed for 6 months after transplantation. Forty-four took a *n-6* PUFA preparation, and 45 the placebo (oleic acid). They found that functional graft survival was significantly better in the *n-6* PUFA group than in those taking the placebo thereby showing the immunosuppressive effects of *n-6* PUFAs. Unfortunately, they also observed an increase in cancer in those receiving the polyunsaturated fats.

Research confirms that transplant recipients are at increased risk of a cancer. The four most common cancers among transplant recipients are non-Hodgkin lymphoma (NHL) and cancers of the lung, kidney, and liver. People with HIV/AIDS (which is a disease of the immune system), also have increased risks of cancers. In both cases, these cancers have been associated with infections, in particular viral infections. NHL can be caused by Epstein-Barr virus infection, and liver cancer by chronic infection with the hepatitis B and hepatitis C viruses.

Further evidence for an immunosuppression and carcinogenesis with vegetable oil is found in a study by Reeve *et al.* where the photo carcinogenic response was measured in hairless mice fed a diet of increasing of polyunsaturated sunflower oil. (**A photo carcinogen is a substance which causes cancer following exposure to radiation**) Six (6) months following the completion of the 10-week chronic UV irradiation treatment, the results show a diet of 20% saturated fat provided almost complete protection, whereas feeding a 20% sunflower oil diet resulted in a 57% reduction in contact hypersensitivity (CHS) reactions. These results provide further evidence that the *n-6* polyunsaturated fat component of the diet induces an immunosuppression which results in an enhancement of photo carcinogenesis.

Studies in humans with a number of inflammatory conditions suggest that both the amount and the type of fat are critical regulators of immune response. The effects on immune function seem to be mediated by both *n-3* and *n-6* unsaturated fatty acids. The *n-6* fatty acids, specifically linoleic, linolenic, and arachidonic acids increase inflammation and immunosuppression through eicosanoids (a family of compounds that are the principal mediators of inflammation we will discuss further later in this chapter), although there is evidence of a direct effect on the cellular components of the immune system as well.

The *n-6* polyunsaturated fats affect both immune cell activation and recruitment, as well as interactions with eicosanoids. Numerous studies have demonstrated that diets high in *n-6* polyunsaturated fat inhibit T-cell responsiveness to stimulation. T-cells are a type of lymphocyte that is intimately involved in the immune response. They are called T-Cells because they originate in the thymus. There are three (3) types of T-cells: *Killer T-cells, Helper T-cells* and *Regulatory T-cells*. Killer T-cells are the cells responsible for locating and destroying foreign particles (like bacteria) and cancerous cells. Helper T-cells modulate the antibody production by B-cells. Regulatory T-cells (Tregs) were first observed in the 1970s. Once activated, Regulatory T-cells target Helper T-cells, blocking their activation and progression of both humoral and cell-mediated immunity.

One possible mechanism for the effect of unsaturated fatty acids on immune cells is by changing the lipid component of the cell membrane. When T-cells are exposed to an invading pathogen, there are marked changes in the membrane phospholipid, fatty acid, and cholesterol composition. Cleland, *et al.*, in 1992 demonstrated the effect of linoleic acid on changes to membrane lipids in an experiment where thirty (30) subjects were randomly allocated into either a high-linoleic acid diet with low saturated fatty acids or a low- linoleic acid, low saturate fat diet. The subjects were observed for a total of seven (7) weeks. Subjects were given a fish-oil supplement at week four (4) and the membrane components of white cells examined. They found that diet alone resulted in a significant change in neutrophil phospholipid. Those subjects on the high-linoleic diet had significantly lower eicosapentaenoic acid (EPA) in neutrophil membranes than the low-linoleic acid group. Clearly, dietary *n-6* fatty acids effects EPA incorporation into neutrophil membranes.

T-regulatory cells are implicated in a number of diseases including disease of autoimmunity, allergy, organ transplant rejection, as well as cancer. In fact, T-reg cells have become an intense area of interest in cancer. These cells are found in relatively high concentrations in tumor draining lymph nodes as well as within the tumor of cancer patients. Many studies have shown that an increase in T-reg cells conferrers a poor prognosis for patients with cancer.

Studies show that reactive oxygen species suppress overall T-cell responses through induction of T-regs, and ROS mediate impairment of T-cell function in cancer patients. The mechanism by which ROS affect T-cell responses still is unclear, but this observation implies that there is an induction of T-reg cells by oxidized unsaturated fatty acids, thereby again linking peroxidation products with cancer.

Another important aspect of immune function influenced by ROS products are the dendritic cells (DC). Dendritic cells are *antigen-presenting cells* whose main function is to attach themselves to antigen material and present it to the T-cells. In other words, DCs are immune cells that locate foreign proteins and present them to T-cells to initiate an immune response. These cells are in constant contact with other cells in the body. DCs origi-

nate in the bone marrow and are typically in an immature state in the peripheral tissues. Upon exposure to
pathogens or inflammation, they undergo a maturation
process. Several studies have shown that oxidized LDL
causes maturation of dendritic cells and are implicated
in atherosclerosis seen in chapter 4.

Multiple studies have demonstrated a marked
dysfunction in dendritic cells in cancer patients. In cancer therapy, antitumor responses depend on functioning of dendritic cells. If the DCs are unable to present
antigens, the T-cells cannot initiate an immune response
to the cancer. It turns out that oxidized lipids block the
cross-presentation of the cancer antigen from DCs to T-
cells! Analysis yields that oxidized-linoleic acid was the
most abundant fatty acid accumulated in dendritic cells.
It is postulated that oxidized lipids reduce the expression of antigens on the cell surface although more research need to be done.

There is an interesting correlation with cholesterol and the three diseases explored so far: immunosuppression, cancer, and coronary heart disease. Those
compounds which inhibit cholesterol synthesis cause a
decreased response of T-lymphocytes. In addition to linoleic and arachidonic acids inhibiting T-cell responses,
cholesterol has a direct effect as well. When 25-hydroxy-
cholesterol (a potent inhibitor of cholesterol synthesis)
is applied to lymphocytes in culture, there is a marked
reduction in activity. The addition of cholesterol to these

cells reverses the effect of 25-hydroxycholesterol and enhances the response of T-cells to pathogens. The presence of cholesterol decreases the fluidity of the membrane and increases killer activity.

A meta-analysis of 23 statin studies with 309,506 person-years of follow-up, demonstrated a significant inverse association between cancer incidence and LDL-C levels. Statins have been shown to be immunosuppressive in clinical studies which may account for their clinical effect as well as the increase in cancer. However, since statins therapy reduces LDL cholesterol levels as well, it is unclear which mechanism is responsible.

The hypothesis as to whether cholesterol is responsible for a decrease in cancer incidence was tested using rats fed either saturated fat to elevate serum cholesterol or 20% safflower oil to minimize serum cholesterol. The rats were then exposed to 1,-2,-dimethylydrazine (DMH) which is known to promote tumor formation. The rats fed the 20% safflower oil diet had significantly greater numbers of large bowel tumors. While the authors surmised that the polyunsaturated diet promoted a decrease in serum cholesterol which in turn augmented tumorigenesis, we know from this and previous chapters that there are other mechanisms by which n-6 polyunsaturated fatty acids can promote carcinogenesis.

Eicosanoids

As mentioned earlier, the immune system is made up of cellular components as well as biochemical messengers. The eicosanoids (from the Greek *eicosa-meaning* "twenty) are twenty (20) carbon fatty acids that circulate in the blood stream and serve to modulate the immune system. In general, the eicosanoids are generated from three polyunsaturated fatty acids:

- Eicosapentaenoic acid (EPA), an n-3 fatty acid with 5 double bonds;
- Arachidonic acid (AA), an n-6 fatty acid, with 4 double bonds;
- Dihomo-gamma-linolenic acid (DGLA), an n-6, with 3 double bonds.

The Eicosanoids are extremely powerful mes-

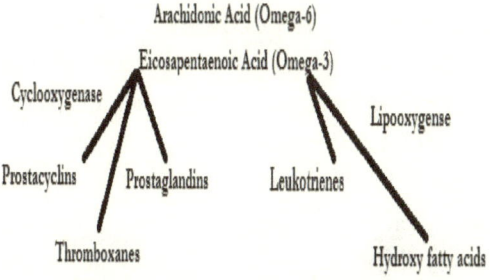

Figure 30: Eicosanoid pathway. n-6 arachidonic is converted via cyclooxygenase to eicosanoids.

sengers, and can be divided into proinflammatory and anti-inflammatory components. The omega-6 polyunsaturated fatty acids are responsible for the pro-inflammatory aspects while the omega-3 polyunsaturated fatty acids are responsible for the anti-inflammatory. Inflammation is a normal response to injury or infection, but when the ratio of n-6 to n-3 polyunsaturated fats is altered, an excessive pro-inflammatory condition exists that results in a wide range of acute and chronic human diseases. Pro-inflammatory diseases are characterized by the production of n-6 eicosanoids such as pro-inflammatory cytokines, arachidonic acid– derived eicosanoids (prostaglandins, thromboxanes, leukotrienes, and other oxidized derivatives), other inflammatory agents (e.g., reactive oxygen species), and adhesion molecules.

Eicosanoids derived from n-3 polyunsaturated fats act as anti-inflammatory agent by replacing arachidonic acid as an eicosanoid substrate and inhibiting arachidonic acid metabolism. Long-chain n-3 polyunsaturated fats also give rise to a family of anti-inflammatory mediators termed <u>resolvins</u>. Evidence from animal studies indicates that resolvins can reduce cellular inflammation by inhibiting the production and transportation of inflammatory cells to the sites of inflammation. Long-chain n-3 polyunsaturated fatty acids found in oily fish and fish oils, also decrease the production of inflammatory eicosanoids, cytokines, and reactive oxygen species and the expression of adhesion molecules.

Fatty acid intake can have profound effects on inflammation and autoimmune disease. Inflammation was first defined by the Roman medic Aulus Cornelius Celsus, in the first century AD, as: *rubor* (redness), *tumor* (swelling), *calor* (heat) and *dolor* (pain). Inflammation is a natural process of elimination of invading pathogens and toxins and to repair damaged tissue. Inflammation is defined by Merriam-Webster as "a local response to cellular injury that is marked by capillary dilatation, leukocyte infiltration, redness, heat, pain, swelling, and often loss of function and that serves as a mechanism initiating the elimination of noxious agents and of damaged tissue."

The clinical response seen in response to excess n-6 polyunsaturated fats is caused by the release of inflammatory mediators, mostly from activated leukocytes that infiltrate into the injured area. Among the key inflammatory mediators are the n-6 eicosanoids, prostaglandin E2 and leukotriene B4, which are derived from n-6 arachidonic acid. The high concentration of n-6 polyunsaturated fats has a profound effect on a large host of diseases, which we will review individually.

Cancer and Inflammation

Rudolf Virchow, the eminent German pathologist and politician, stated in 1865 that the cause of cancer was inflammation caused by white blood cells. Although this concept has long been suspected, inflammation as the cause for cancer has been largely ignored, and only recently has this hypothesis been confirmed. Microscopic analysis of invasive breast carcinomas indicate that leukocytes can account for as much 50% of the total tumor mass. Historically, these tumor-infiltrating leukocytes (TILs) have been considered to be the result of the immune system mounting a failed attempt to launch an immunological attack on the tumor. However, there is increasing evidence that the leukocyte infiltration actually promotes tumor angiogenesis, growth and tissue invasion. This may be the result of inflammatory cells secreting n-6 pro-inflammatory eicosanoids which stimulate proliferation and invasiveness of cancer cells.

Clinical data on solid tumors show a correlation between high-density leukocyte infiltration into tumors and poor outcome of patients with cancers of different origins. It is clear that several inflammatory markers are expressed in various cancers and mediate their progression. Therefore, those compounds which suppress these inflammatory markers have a potential for prevention and treatment of cancer.

One such compound is aspirin. Figure 30 shows how cyclooxygenase (COX) enzymes (i.e., COX-1 and COX-2) catalyze the conversion of n-6 arachidonic acid into prostaglandin (PG). PG is further metabolized into different PGs, including PGE2, PGD2, PGF2, PGI2 and thromboxane. Aspirin is the only drug that is able to permanently inhibit COX-1 and COX-2 activity. COX-2 expression is upregulated in 40%–50% of human colorectal adenomas and in 80%–90% of carcinomas! COX-2 plays a pivotal role in tumor initiation, promotion and progression by increasing n-6 eicosanoids and reactive oxygen species (ROS).

Numerous clinical studies support the role of COX-2 in cancer. A meta-analysis published in *The Lancet*, analyzed patient records from 51 trials that compared people who took aspirin every day to people who took no aspirin. They found that taking daily low-dose aspirin (less than 300 mg) for 3 years resulted in approximately a 25% lowered risk of developing any type of cancer.

Another study published in *The Lancet* looked at the effect of aspirin on cancer metastasis (spread). Those cancer patients taking aspirin (75mg or more a day), lowered their risk of metastatic cancer by 36%. A sub analysis of the data revealed that metastatic adenocarcinoma (a solid tumor, including colon, lung, and prostate), accounted for a reduction of 46%! In addition, daily aspirin lowered the risk of non-metastatic cancer progressing to metastatic cancer. The lower risk of metastatic cancer with aspirin was confirmed in *The Lancet Oncology*. The authors found significantly lowered risk of cancer and metastasis in colon, throat, gastric, biliary and breast cancer.

Other research has suggested a similar link between aspirin and prevention of other types of cancer. A 2011 study in The Lancet, for example, found that taking at least 75 milligrams of aspirin per day, over the course of five years, significantly reduced the risk of colon cancer.

One of the more compelling evidence for the cancer prevention effects of aspirin comes from nine non-cancer clinical trials, representing data from >23,000 patients. The meta-analysis of these studies demonstrated nearly 20% decreased risk in overall cancer mortality after a 20-year follow-up period, with most of the benefit occurring after five years of aspirin. The reduction of cancers was most significant for esophageal and colorectal cancers.

In another meta-analysis involving 51 trials (representing ~77,500 patients), daily aspirin versus no aspirin was evaluated for cancer deaths. Aspirin reduced the risk of cancer death and colorectal cancer and lymphoma. The aspirin benefit occurred after 5 years of follow-up. Further, aspirin appeared to reduce the metastatic spread of adenocarcinoma.

CaPSURE (Cancer of the Prostate Strategic Urologic Research Endeavor), study of approximately 15,000 men with all stages of biopsy-proven prostate cancer. Patients have enrolled at 43 community urology practices, academic medical centers, and VA hospitals throughout the United States since 1995. Researchers looked at nearly 6,000 men who had localized prostate cancer. Just over one-third of the men, or 2,175 of the 5,955, were taking anticoagulants, mostly aspirin. The prostate cancer death rate for those taking aspirin was 3 percent, compared with 8 percent for those who did not over the 10-year period. In other words, the death rate was reduced by over 60%! The aspirin users were also significantly less likely to experience a recurrence of prostate cancer or have the disease spread to the bones.

Researchers at the Fox Chase Cancer Center in Philadelphia reported that among 2,051 prostate cancer patients they followed, those not using aspirin were twice as likely to experience a recurrence of prostate cancer within 18 months, as detected by rising scores on the prostate-specific antigen test (PSA).

In summary, n-6 polyunsaturated fats modulate the immune system affecting both cellular and eicosanoids components. The typical Western diet contains 20 to 25-fold more n-6 fats than n-3 fats resulting in a pro-inflammatory state. This pro-inflammatory state is observed in cancer and other immune diseases including arthrosclerosis. It is clear from aspirin studies that inhibiting cyclooxygenase (COX) results in a reduction of cancer and cancer metastases. It would be very interesting to see what the cumulative effect would be of eliminating n-6 polyunsaturated fat (vegetable oils) and aspirin on cancer outcome.

7. Obesity and Diabetes

There has been an alarming increase in obesity and its associated co-morbidities in the United States since the introduction of vegetable oil in the American diet. There are estimates that suggest approximately 36% of the U.S. population is currently obese and by 2030 this will increase to over 50% (Figure 31).

The increase in obesity closely correlates with consumption of polyunsaturated fats (Figure 32). By now, you should suspect that obesity is linked to a wide array of pathophysiologic conditions including metabolic syndrome, insulin resistance, type 2 diabetes, hypertension, hyperlipidemia, cancer, and atherosclerosis.

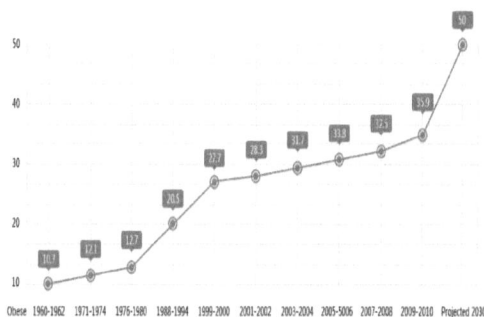

Figure 31: Prevalence of obesity among adults in the United States ages 20-74.

In fact, you might consider obesity, metabolic syndrome, insulin resistance and type 2 diabetes as the same disease, just different stages in the downward progression of the condition. In this chapter, we will explore the role of dietary fats on the maintenance of body weight and the development of co-morbidities.

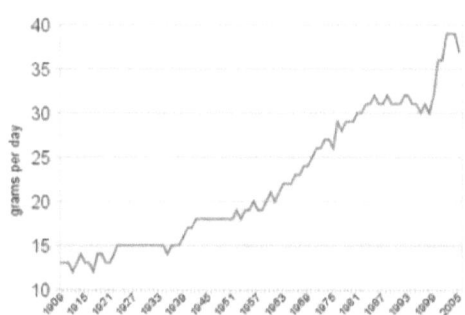

Figure 32: Consumption of polyunsaturated fat in the United States from 1909-2005.

Regulation of body weight is an extremely complex physiological mechanism that would require an entire book to cover adequately. We simply marvel at the absolute efficiency in which we consume a meal that must be digested and stored within a few hours! Day in and day out. Body weight is effectively maintained during periods of plenty and fasting. This requires a coordination of cellular components, multiple hormones, and behavioral input from the brain. It is only when we introduce foods that were not part of the evolutionary history do we throw a wrench in the mechanisms. To stay focused on the problems of vegetable oils, we will focus on those areas where polyunsaturated fats play a role in weight dysfunction: mitochondrial function, immunological-inflammatory causes, leptin resistance, adiponectin levels, and insulin resistance.

Mitochondrial Function (Dysfunction)

We previous examined the role of the mitochondria in cancer and how polyunsaturated fats modify the function of the mitochondrial membranes. Therefore, we should expect the same changed in mitochondrial function would be implicated in obesity. And indeed, the seems to be the case.

Throughout the literature there is reference to "age related" decline in mitochondrial function. We all know too well that maintenance of an ideal body weight becomes far more difficult as we age. There are many theories for this, but it is obvious that our mitochondria do not function the same as when we were young.

If we look at a baby's mitochondria, the fat composition of his/her cardiolipin is mostly palmitic acid, a saturated fatty acid. But as we age, the palmitic acid in the mitochondrial cardiolipin is replaced by polyunsaturated fats from the diet. The changes to the molecular configuration of cardiolipin causes the mitochondria to becomes unstable with increasing polyunsaturated incorporation. This instability disrupts the critical function of cytochrome oxidase leading to a decline in function. The replacement of palmitic acid with polyunsaturated fats corresponds to the life-long decline of the person's metabolic rate known as "age related". This decline in function means we can't metabolize efficiently, therefore fats that can't be metabolized are stored in adipose tissue.

Cytochrome c oxidase (or complex IV) is a large protein found in the inner membrane of the mitochondria and is part of the electron transport system. The electron transport chain is a group of compounds that pass electrons from one to another across the mitochondrial membrane ultimately transferring electrons to oxygen. Four membrane-bound complexes have been identified in mitochondria. Each is an extremely complex structure that is embedded in the inner membrane. The function of respiratory complexes I and IV are significantly decreased with age in old rats (26-33 month of age) compared to the activity of the same enzymes in young animals.

The fatty acid composition of the mitochondria of old rats differed from that of young animals by a decreased content of myristic, oleic, linoleic, and α-linolenic acids and enhanced content of dihomo-γ-linolenic, arachidonic, and docosahexaenoic acids. When hydrogenated peanut oil is added of the diet of the older rat, the functional capability of complex IV is completely restored as well as 80% of complex I. The fatty acid contents are reversed as well, indicating the changes in the electron transport system seen in aging are reversible.

The observation of fatty acid content between older mitochondria and those in younger animals has been repeated in other studies, thereby demonstrating that cardiolipin remodeling occurs with aging, specifically with an increase in highly unsaturated fatty acids. In one experiment, rats were given either a diet high in saturated fat (coconut oil) or linoleic acid (polyunsaturated n-6 18:2). Basal respiration was significantly increased by in the animals fed coconut oil.

As we saw in cancer, peroxidized polyunsaturated fats disrupts mitochondrial function. The same holds true for reactive oxygen species on the activities of the electron transport chain. Reactive oxygen species causes a peroxidation of cardiolipin which affects the activity of cytochrome c oxidase. If new cardiolipin is added, there is an almost complete restoration of the ROS-induced loss of cytochrome c oxidase activity. However, no restoration was obtained with peroxidized cardiolipin.

Reactive products of lipid peroxidation, especially 4-hydroxynonenal (HNE), play an important role in the decreased mitochondrial membrane fluidity observed in aging. Both 4-hydroxynonenal (HNE) and malondialdehyde (MDA) decreases membrane fluidity in the mitochondria. It seems likely that lipid peroxidation product modifies the membrane fluidity by direct interaction with membrane phospholipids.

Malondialdehyde causes a dose-dependent inhibition of mitochondrial complex I- and complex II. In addition, MDA significantly elevates mitochondrial reactive oxygen species (ROS). So, in addition to increasing membrane fluidity and peroxidation of cardiolipin, peroxidized polyunsaturated fats causes mitochondrial dysfunction by directly promoting generation of ROS and thereby modifying mitochondrial proteins.

Mitochondrial abnormalities have also been reported in both type 2 diabetes and insulin-resistant states. Diabetes, as in obesity, is also associated with damage caused by reactive oxygen species, leading to mitochondrial and cellular oxidative damage. This contributes to the development and progression of diabetic complications. We will discuss the underlying mechanism type 2 diabetes and its relation to obesity later in this chapter.

Insulin Resistance

Insulin is a hormone produced in the beta cell in the pancreas. Insulin release is stimulated by either glucose or protein. Following a meal, insulin levels increase to facilitate the movement of glucose into cells and thereby keeping glucose levels low.

- Insulin stimulates the incorporation of glucose into muscle, fat, and liver cells

- Insulin stimulates the liver and muscle tissue to store excess glucose as glycogen.

- Insulin also lowers blood glucose levels by reducing glucose production in the liver.

An important role of insulin is in the regulation of lipids. Insulin decreases the rate of fat breakdown or lipolysis in adipose tissue and thereby lowers the plasma fatty acid level. Insulin stimulates fatty acid and triacylglycerol synthesis in tissues; increases the uptake of triglycerides from the blood into adipose tissue and muscle; and decreases the rate of fatty acid oxidation in muscle and liver.

Glucagon is a peptide hormone, produced by alpha cells of the pancreas, that raises the concentration of glucose in the bloodstream. Its effect is opposite that of insulin. Glucagon is also known to cause the release of free fatty acids from adipose tissue.

In short, the fat cell is controlled by the actions of the two opposing hormones. When a meal is consumed, insulin is released from the pancreas and binds to the insulin receptor on the fat cell thereby activating the glucose transporter to take up the excess blood glucose into the cell. In addition, insulin stimulates lipogenesis and blocks lipolysis. In-between meals, or with fasting, insulin levels decline and glucagon levels increase to maintain blood glucose levels. In addition, lipolysis is increased causing fatty acids to be released.

We have somehow been entrained to eat three meals per day. With consumption of breakfast, there is a rapid spike in insulin followed by a show decline over the next several hours. The insulin levels decline just in time for lunch when insulin spikes again and then slowly decline. The same is repeated at dinner. So, for most of the waking period, insulin levels are elevated and fat cells are lipogenesis mode. Add snacking to the mix and you have a recipe for insulin resistance (Figure 33).

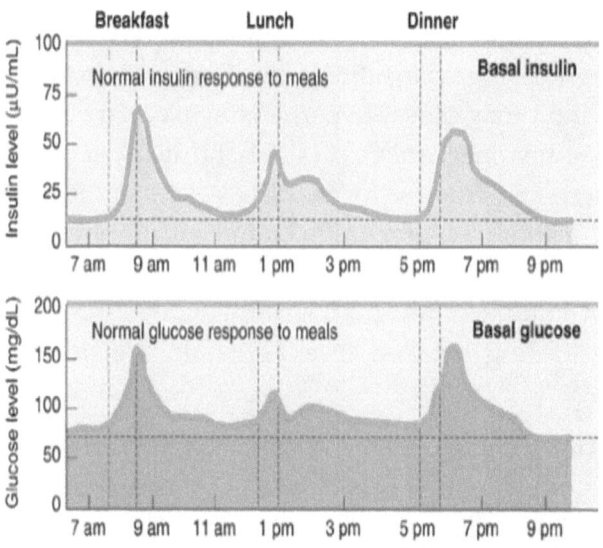

Figure 33: Insulin and glucose daily rollercoaster.

In 1998, Barnard *et al.* showed that a high-fat re-fined-sugar diet mimicking the western diet caused insulin resistance in rats. The insulin resistance and hyper-insulinemia occur be-fore the other manifestations of the metabolic syndrome showing that diet, and not obesity, is the underlying cause.

Fructose has been implicated in the development of insulin resistance. Fructose is not metabolized via the same pathways as glucose. Instead fructose is shunted to the liver leading to rapid stimulation of lipogenesis, triglyceride formation, and lipoprotein formation as discussed previously. Triglyceride accumulation contributes to reduced insulin sensitivity and hepatic insulin resistance/glucose intolerance. While fructose does not increase insulin levels, chronic exposure to fructose indirectly causes hyperinsulinemia and obesity through other mechanisms. Litherland *et al.* showed feeding rats 66% fructose for two (2) weeks, significantly lowered insulin receptor mRNA, and insulin receptor numbers in both skeletal muscle and liver compared to rats fed a standard chow diet. Twenty-eight (28) days of fructose feeding resulted in a 72% reduction insulin function.

The increased demand for insulin requires an over production of insulin by the beta cells in the pancreas (Figure 34). As long as the beta cells are able to produce enough

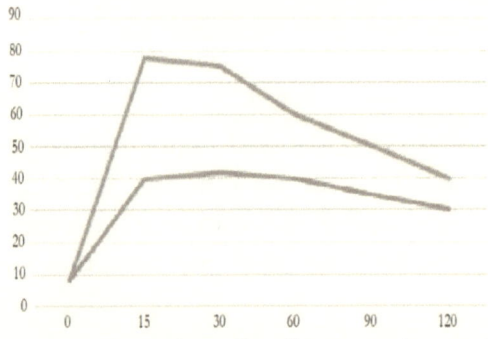

Figure 34: Comparison of insulin response in normal and obese individuals.

insulin to overcome the insulin resistance, a state called metabolic syndrome exists. Over time though, as the beta cells decline, type 2 diabetes can develop. Metabolic syndrome is a cluster of symptoms including increased blood pressure, a high blood sugar level, excess body fat around the waist and abnormal cholesterol levels.

A link between an increase in dietary n-6 polyunsaturated fats and the development of insulin resistance was shown in a study where mice were fed corn oil for 6 weeks. The corn-oil fed mice demonstrated reduced locomotor activity, accompanied by a lower respiratory ratio, hyperinsulinemia, and impaired glucose metabolism. The skeletal muscle of these mice failed to up-regulate fat oxidation genes, thereby supporting the metabolic insufficiencies observed in these mice.

Fortunately, weight loss usually reverses insulin resistance. Also, increasing the fasting periods will allow for more recovery time for the pancreas and allowing lipolysis in adipose tissue because of the declining insulin levels.

Immunological-Inflammatory Causes of Obesity

As we have seen in the diseases examined so far, there is a correlation with obesity and cancer, heart disease, and diabetes. The search for a unifying mechanism behind obesity and in co-morbidities has led to the discovery that obesity is an immune disease. More evidence has emerged that inflammation is involved in the development of insulin resistance. There is also evidence of increased inflammatory eicosanoid production and increased inflammation in skeletal muscle, adipose tissue as well as pancreas islet cells in obesity.

The notion that adipose tissue is simply a storage mechanism for fat has changed with the observation that fat cells produce inflammatory eicosanoids. In obese patients, a chronic low-grade inflammation exists with increased plasma levels of C-reactive protein, and inflammatory eicosanoids such as Tumor Necrosis Factor (TNF), Interluekin-6 (IL-6), Interluekin-8 (IL-8), and Monocyte Chemoattractant Protein-1 (MCP-1). It has been estimated that there is an <u>excess</u> of 20–30 million macrophages with each kilogram of excess fat in humans. MCP-1 stimulates the recruitment of macrophages into adipose tissue. Therefore, by virtue of the increase in fat mass in the obese individual, it is no surprise that and inflammatory state exists in obesity.

In addition to inflammatory eicosanoid production in adipose tissue, there is also evidence of increased eicosanoid production with inflammation in skeletal muscle in obese individuals. The muscle in the obese individual also has infiltrating macrophages similar to what is seen in adipose tissue. There is also evidence of inflammation in pancreatic islets, triggering beta cell apoptosis with a reduction in insulin secretion and a progression to diabetes.

There is mounting evidence suggesting a mechanism between inflammation and adipose tissue that is located within certain tissues, such as the colon, lymph nodes, myocardium, and large arteries. Activated adipocytes generate eicosanoids that contribute to the inflammatory response in organs where the adipose tissue resides. For example, a relationship has been proposed between cardiac adipose tissue and heart disease. Increased macrophage accumulation in adipose tissue around the heart may account for the enhanced inflammatory potential.

As we saw in the previous chapter on immunity, dietary fats can have a modulating effect on the inflammatory process. TLRs are a class of protein receptors usually expressed in sentinel cells such as macrophages and dendritic cells. These receptors recognize molecules on microbes, which activate immune cell responses. Elevated levels of TLR-4 have been reported in the obese individuals on the insulin target tissues such as liver, muscle, brain, adipose tissue, vasculature, and pancreatic β-cells. TRLs signal the immune cells to produce the inflammatory eicosanoids which trigger inflammation.

Omega-3 EPA and DHA were found to inhibit the TLR-4 pathway. These findings suggest that EPA and DHA may reduce the secretion of pro-inflammatory cytokines, and prevent macrophage infiltration into adipose tissue.

With the increase of per capita consumption of vegetable oils, we can assume that fats stored in adipose tissue would reflect this increase. And this is indeed the case. The percentage of linoleic acid stored in body fat rose over 200 percent from 1960 to 2008 as seen in Figure 35. Therefore, studies that look at dietary effects of polyunsaturated fats on obesity would be suspect, in the short term, due to the high amounts of n-6 fats in adipose tissue.

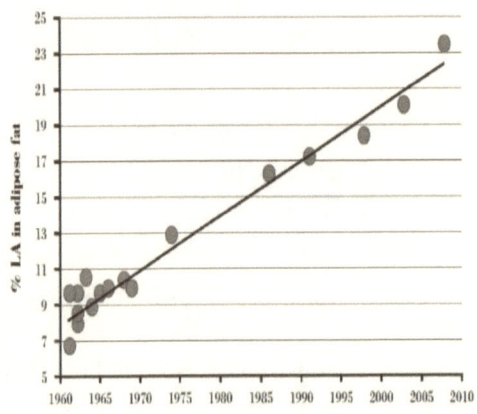

Figure 35: Changes in Linoleic Acid content in body fat from 1961 to 2008 – United States.

Instead of looking at dietary consumption of polyunsaturated fat and its effect on obesity, we can instead look at the peroxidation of PUFAs in the form of their oxidation end product Malondialdehyde (MDA) and 4-hydroxy-nonenal (HNE). MDA as discussed earlier is an important indicator of lipid peroxidation that is generated as an end product from oxidative degradation of n-6 polyunsaturated fatty acids.

Several studies have confirmed that the concentration of serum malondialdehyde increases with increasing BMI. Obese individuals exhibit a higher level of serum malondialdehyde as compared to normal-weight subjects. In contrast, cellular antioxidant super-oxide dismutase (SOD) and glutathione peroxidase are significantly decreased in the obese individuals. This increase in oxidative stress is correlated with serum leptin level and BMI suggesting MDA overwhelms the internal cellular defenses against ROS formation.

Studies have demonstrated that MDA can induce potent inflammatory cytokine expression in macrophages as well as peripheral blood monocytes and augmented expression seen in peripheral blood monocytes from diabetic patients. MDA induces significant increases in 47 key pro-inflammatory molecules.

4-HNE, which is also derived from peroxidation of n-6 polyunsaturated fatty acids such as arachidonic and linoleic acids, is one of the most abundant and active lipid peroxides in obesity. From previous chapters we know that 4-HME forms stable adducts with proteins, thereby modulating cellular activities. High levels of 4-HNE induce apoptosis in fat cells, whereas lower concentrations can act as a growth regulating factor by modulating cell growth and differentiation. 4-HME can damage pancreatic β cells and can impair the ability of muscle and liver cells to respond to insulin. Like MDA, 4-HNE also alters cellular responses including inflammatory response, protein degradation, mitochondria function, and insulin signaling.

Similar to MDA, levels of HNE are increased in the blood and muscle tissue of obese subjects compared to normal weight subjects. Improved insulin sensitivity in muscle cells resulting from exercise or dietary energy restriction is associated with reduced levels of HNE and other n-6 polyunsaturated peroxidation products.

Leptin

Leptin is a hormone secreted by white adipocytes. Leptin levels are highly correlated with the total amount of white fat in the body. Leptin functions by binding to hypothalamic receptors in the brain which in turn modifies food intake through suppression of appetite. Leptin therefore acts as a negative feedback loop to regulate body weight. Increased body fat means more leptin which in turn lowers food intake inducing a feeling of satiety.

Leptin also increases insulin sensitivity in rats. Therefore, a decrease in leptin contributes to insulin resistance. Leptin increases free fatty acid oxidation in mouse muscle by 42%, whereas insulin decreases fatty acid oxidation by 40%. Leptin inhibits insulin biosynthesis and secretion from the pancreatic β-cells. In turn, insulin stimulates leptin secretion from adipose tissue, establishing a hormonal regulatory feedback loop. A leptin resistance can lead to an increase in insulin secretion, which in turn decreases lipolysis in adipose tissue contributing to obesity and insulin resistance.

Several hormones can modulate leptin secretion, the most important of these are insulin and norepinephrine. Studies have shown that insulin acutely stimulates leptin secretion and that norepinephrine, exert a strong inhibitory effect on insulin-stimulated leptin secretion.

Starvation or fasting decreases plasma leptin concentrations in adipose tissue as well.

Evidence indicates that the consumption of a diet high in n-6 polyunsaturated fatty acids is associated with the development of leptin resistance and obesity. Further, it has been demonstrated that n-6 polyunsaturated fatty acid intake directly influences adipose tissue secretion of leptin. Also, arachidonic acid attenuates the effect of leptin on hepatic glucose and lipid metabolism, as well as diminishes the glucose transporter, lipogenesis and cholesterol synthesis. These results indicate that an increased dietary consumption to n-6 PUFA induces leptin resistance!

Adiponectin

Adiponectin is a protein hormone secreted from adipose tissue that regulates a number of metabolic processes, including glucose regulation and fatty acid oxidation. Adiponectin is known to enhance insulin sensitivity and to act as an anti-inflammatory agent as well as an anti-atherogenic effects which appears to protect against arteriosclerosis. As such, lower levels of adiponectin have been implicated in the insulin resistance and pro-inflammatory states associated with obesity. Insulin resistance and obesity causes lower plasma adiponectin concentrations. Low levels of adiponectin expression have also been observed in the visceral fat of diabetic rats in comparison with lean rats.

Adiponectin receptors are ubiquitous appearing

in higher concentration in muscle and liver. The primary mechanisms by which adiponectin enhance insulin sensitivity appears to be through increased fatty acid oxidation and inhibition of glucose production in the liver. In contrast, adiponectin levels are reduced by pro-inflammatory cytokines especially tumor necrosis factor.

In addition, adiponectin is involved in preventing arthrosclerosis by inhibiting monocyte adhesion to endothelial cells, macrophage transformation to foam cells, and vascular smooth muscle cell proliferation. In a mouse model of atherosclerosis, increasing adiponectin expression reduced atherosclerotic lesions. In another mouse study, mice that were adiponectin-deficient exhibit exaggerated vascular remodeling as well as diet-induced insulin resistance. Therefore, adiponectin has potential in modulating arthrosclerosis in addition to anti-diabetic properties.

In mice, changes in adipose tissue content of 4-HNE causes a decline in plasma adiponectin. The decrease in adiponectin secretion is dose-dependent with 4-HNE levels in the adipocytes. In contrast, adiponectin gene expression is significantly elevated. It has been shown that 4-HNE acts through an increase in adiponectin degradation. Findings from human and rodent studies suggest the production of adiponectin increases with dietary intake of EPA and DHA. In summary, peroxidation end products of n-6 polyunsaturated fats play a direct role in obesity-related plasma adiponectin decline and may contribute to type 2 diabetes and arthrosclerosis as well.

In summary, dietary vegetable oils combined with sugar and high fructose creates the prefect storm for obesity, ultimately leading to type II diabetes. Multiple feedings of these dietary elements, without adequate periods of fasting, leads to insulin resistance that causes a spectrum of diseases from obesity, metabolic syndrome to diabetes. Contributing to this mix is the effect of polyunsaturated fats and their peroxidation products causing a decline in adiponectin levels, induction of leptin resistance, and an increase in inflammatory eicosanoids. Fortunately, much of this is reversible!

8. Diet Modification

Hopefully, by this point, you have been convinced that seed oils are impacting your health. And one would believe that elimination of seed oils from you diet would be as easy as throwing out all "vegetable oils". Unfortunately, it is not so easy. Seed oils are widely used in an astonishingly large number of products. For example, salad dressings are little more than flavored soybean oil! By definition, mayonnaise is 60% vegetable oil. Canola, corn, safflower, cotton seed oil and soybean oil are found in soups, margarines, peanut butter, ice cream, even baby formula. You wouldn't think of eating cotton seed oil, but there it is in peanut butter.

Elimination of seed oils from the diet is not something that can be done in moderation. To successfully stop and hopefully reverse, the health consequence from vegetable oils, you must eliminate as much of the omega-6 fatty acids from the diet as possible. This means you need to focus carefully on the label. To start:

- Any vegetable oil (except olive, avocado, or coconut) – throw it out

- Any margarine – throw it out

- Any oil based salad dressing – throw it out

- Any peanut butter – throw it out

- Any fried snack including potato chips – throw it out

- Spaghetti sauce, if it contains seed oils – throw it out

- Any fried food – throw it out.

You begin get the whole picture when looking at the food label and realizing how ubiquitous these oils have become in our diet over a relatively short period of time.

This may, at first, appear as a drastic change in your dietary habits, but there are substitutes. Firstly, olive and avocado oils are Ok as long as they are used in moderation and are not heated. These are mono-saturated fats so they will form peroxidation products with heating. An alternative to vegetable oils is coconut oil. It is primarily a saturated fat so it will not oxidize. Coconut oil is gaining in popularity and there are many testimonials to the benefit of switching to coconut oil. If you purchase refined coconut oil, it will not have the coconut flavor found in many unrefined oils.

Use butter instead of margarine. Real butter, especially from grass fed animals, tastes much better anyway. Look at the label for margarine and compare it to butter. Instead of seed oils, flavorings, coloring, preservatives, etc., butter simply contains cream and salt.

Salad dressing used to be yogurt based. Some still are but you need to look for them in the refrigerated section of your supermarket. Alternatively, use oil and vinegar. There are many recipes for salad dressings that use buttermilk or yogurt as a base instead of oil.

Stored omega-6 fats

Elimination of dietary omega 6 fatty acids is only the first step. There are still the years of accumulated omega 6 fats stored in body fat to deal with. There is no easy way to do this except to reduce the fat content of adipose tissue.

Depending on your age, you have been accumulating omega-6 fats during your life time. To reverse the health effect of vegetable oils, these need to be removed from your fat stores by stimulating lipolysis. From the previous discussion on obesity, we know that lipolysis is dependent on hormone-sensitive lipase. And lipase is modulated by insulin levels.

Conventional diets don't work. And "low glycemic" or "low carbohydrate" diets fail due to a simple inconvenient fact. That fact is proteins elevate insulin levels! Look at the following table. The glucose (or glycemic) score is the percentage change in blood glucose levels relative to white bread. The insulin score is the percent change in insulin levels relative to white bread.

As expected carbohydrates increase blood glucose levels with a corresponding increase in insulin. But look at proteins. As early as 1915, it has been known that amino acids present in dietary proteins could be used by the body to produce glucose. For most common proteins, 50–80 g of glucose can be derived from 100 g of ingested protein! For example, subjects who ate 50 grams of cottage cheese protein produced 9.7 g of carbohydrate. This in part explains why lean fish consumption is positively associated with type II diabetes.

Take a look at cheese. Cheese has the capacity to raise insulin levels on average by 45%. However, if you standardize the corresponding insulin increase by the weight of food ingested, then cheese raises insulin by staggering 106%. This means cheese is able to increase insulin weight-by-weight more than pasta, rice, or French fries, putting it on par with ice cream!

I am not suggesting by any means that you curtail protein in the diet. To the contrary, a continuous protein source is essential. I am making two points. Low carbohydrate diets fail in part, because of the misinformation that proteins do not stimulate insulin.

More importantly, it is not what we eat, so much

Food	Food Category	Glucose Score%	Insulin Index %	Insulin per gm serving weight
	Cereal			
All-Bran		40 ± 7	32 ± 4	25 ± 3
Special K		70 ± 9	66 ± 5	47 ± 4
Corn Flakes		76 ± 11	75 ± 8	52 ± 4
	Carbohydrates			
White Pasta		46 ± 10	40 ± 5	22 ± 2
Grain Bread		60 ± 12	56 ± 6	62 ± 8
White Rice		110 ± 15	79 ± 12	40 ± 3
Potatoes		141 ± 35	121 ± 11	38 ± 4
French Fries		71 ± 16	74 ± 12	82 ± 8
Baked Beans		114 ± 18	120 ± 19	57 ± 11
	Protein			
Eggs		42 ± 16	31 ± 6	30 ± 6
Cheese		55 ± 18	45 ± 13	106 ± 27
Beef		21 ± 8	51 ± 16	37 ± 9
Fish		28 ± 13	59 ± 18	28 ± 6
	Fruit			
Apples		50 ± 6	59 ± 4	20 ± 2
Oranges		39 ± 7	60 ± 3	15 ± 2
Grapes		74 ± 9	82 ± 6	31 ± 3
Bananas		79 ± 10	81 ± 5	45 ± 5
	Snacks			
Peanuts		12 ± 4	20 ± 5	88 ± 22
Popcorn		52 ± 9	54 ± 9	139 ± 14
Potato Chips		52 ± 9	61 ± 14	186 ± 36
Ice Cream		70 ± 9	89 ± 13	103 ± 16
Yogurt		62 ± 15	115 ± 13	65 ± 7
	Baked Goods			
Donuts		63 ± 12	74 ± 9	191 ± 37
Croissants		74 ± 9	79 ± 14	215 ± 47
Crackers		118 ± 24	87 ± 12	253 ± 46
Cookies		74 ± 11	92 ± 15	298 ± 75
Cakes		56 ± 14	82 ± 12	223 ± 54
White Bead		100 ± 0	100 ± 0	187 ± 33

Figure 36: Changes in glycemic score and change in insulin following eating certain foods.

as when we eat it. I will explain later.

Incretin

In the mid-1960's a number of groups showed that glucose, given orally, induced a greater insulin response than glucose given intravenously. This confirmed the hypothesis, which was first postulated in 1902 by Bayliss and Starling, that oral glucose induces release of "incretins" into the bloodstream. In 1971, John C. Brown isolated and subsequently determined the structure of a peptide he had isolated from intestinal mucosa. Administration of the peptide inhibited gastric acid secretion in dogs, so he called it gastric inhibitory polypeptide (GIP)1. Brown and colleagues subsequently found that it had insulinotropic (insulin stimulating) properties and suggested that it be called glucose dependent insulinotropic peptide, retaining the acronym GIP. They not only demonstrated that GIP elevates insulin, but also demonstrated that plasma glucose must be elevated in order for GIP to induce insulin secretion.

Incretins are hormones that are released from the gut into the bloodstream in response to ingestion of food, and they then modulate the insulin secretory response. The insulin secretory response of incretins, called the incretin effect, accounts for at least 50% of the total insulin secreted after oral glucose.

Carr, *et al.* in 2008 published the results of their study entitled *Incretin and Islet Hormonal Responses to Fat and Protein Ingestion in Healthy Men.* This study examined incretin and insulin hormone responses to ingestion of pure fat or protein over 5 hours in healthy men, using plain water ingestion as the control.

Both fat and protein ingestion increased insulin, glucagon, GIP, and GLP-1 levels without affecting glucose levels. This was associated with seven-fold higher insulin and glucagon responses compared with fat ingestion (Figure 37). Looking at Figure 38, we see the incretin (GLP-1) effect is rapid and prolonged over 240 minutes. In other words, consuming protein will increase insulin levels that do not return to fasting levels for four hours.

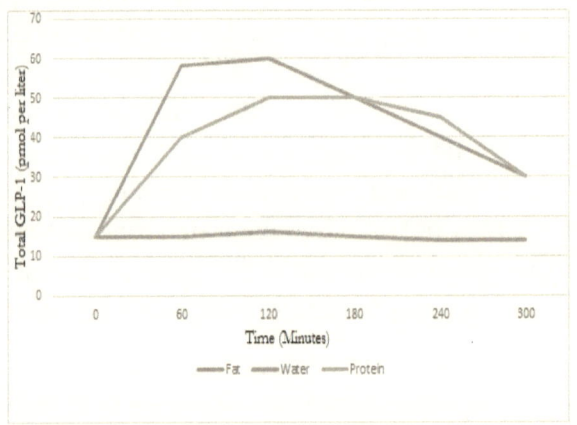

Figure 37: Total incretin (GLP-1), before and during 300 min after ingestion of fat, protein, or water in healthy male volunteers.

Both fat and protein ingestion increases GLP-1 levels (Figure 38). The GLP-1 response is similar after protein and fat ingestion. GLP-1 levels remain elevated throughout the 300-minute test period.

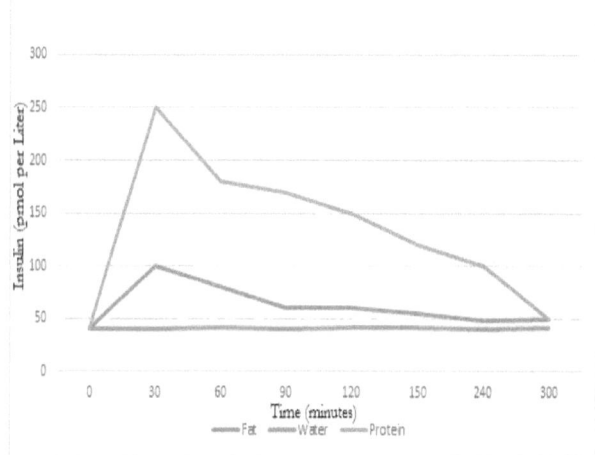

Figure 38: Plasma levels of insulin, before and during 300 min after ingestion of fat, protein, or water in healthy male volunteers.

In summary, the gut is the largest endocrine organ in the body, releasing incretin following ingestion of proteins and fats that, in turn, increases insulin levels. This is important not only in understanding of why low carbohydrate diets fail, and but also understanding the proper way to diet.

Growth Hormone

From numerous studies in humans, it is clear that growth hormone (GH) is negatively associated with adipose tissue, and improves overall body mass by increasing fat catabolism as well as protein anabolism. As evidence, individuals with GH deficiency have an increased fat mass, and treatment of their GH deficiency with GH reverses the fat mass increase. Bengtsson, *et al.*

found that GH treatment in individuals with GH deficiency reduced total body fat by 9.4%, abdominal adipose tissue by 30%, and subcutaneous adipose tissue by 13%. Johannsson *et al.* reported similar results in GH deficient patients. They found a reduction in total body fat (9.2%) with abdominal fat reduced to a higher degree (18.1%) than subcutaneous adipose tissue (6.1%).

GH administration also induces hepatic LDL receptors two-fold, with a resultant decrease in serum cholesterol by 25%. The LDL receptor stimulation is of a similar magnitude as seen in cholesterol lowering drugs. This suggests that GH has an important role in the regulation plasma LDL levels in humans as well.

Different dietary elements have opposite effects on GH release. For example, glucose and fatty acids suppress GH release, while certain amino acids stimulate secretion. One of the most potent hormones that stimulates GH release is *ghrelin*. Ghrelin is produced in the stomach. When the stomach is empty, ghrelin is secreted, and when the stomach is stretched, secretion stops. Ghrelin is also known as the hunger hormone and acts on brain cells in the hypothalamus to increase hunger, and to increase gastric acid secretion. In fasting conditions, ghrelin is released which in turn stimulates GH production.

Eating three meals a day does not allow for stomach emptying therefore creating a perpetual state of GH deficiency. Fasting is an effective means to increase GH levels and decrease adipose tissue mass. Kian, *et al.*, in 1987 looked at six individuals over a five day fast. The subjects lost an average of 10.5 lbs. during the five days of fasting. There was a progressive fall in blood glucose. Fasting also resulted in a progressive increase in GH. However, eating carbohydrates causes a rapid reversal of fasting metabolism.

Taking what we have learned here, it is not so much what you eat as when you eat it. Fasting raises GH levels and decreases glucose and insulin levels. This creates an environment that favors lipolysis thereby reducing adipose tissue mass. Although five days of fasting might be considered impossible, fasting for shorter periods (i.e. 24 hrs.) is common for our pets, and no doubt primitive man found himself in a frequent fasting state as he foraged for food. Eating three meals a day, no matter the calorie restriction or food type, is counterproductive and doomed to failure. Unless counter-indicated, fasting for 20-24 hrs., or some other form of intermittent fasting will ultimately reduce body fat with the added benefit of breaking insulin resistance and improving cholesterol profiles.

Carbohydrates

There has been much discussion on the topic of carbohydrates and their role in the diet without much attention on the differences in carbohydrate structure. Like fats, there are differences in carbohydrate structures that results in differences in the way the sugars are metabolized. Carbohydrates are, as its name implies, "hydrates" of carbon atoms. This means carbohydrates consist of carbon atoms bound to hydrogen and oxygen at a 2:1 ratio which is the same ratio as water (H_2O). Carbohydrates are also known as saccharides from the Greek, meaning "sugar". The names of sugars often contain the suffix -ose. Most sugars found in nature exist as disaccharides (two)or polysaccharides (many). For example, cane sugar is a disaccharide consisting of glucose and fructose. Milk sugar or lactose is the pairing of galactose and glucose, while maltose is the combination of two glucose molecules (see Figure 39).

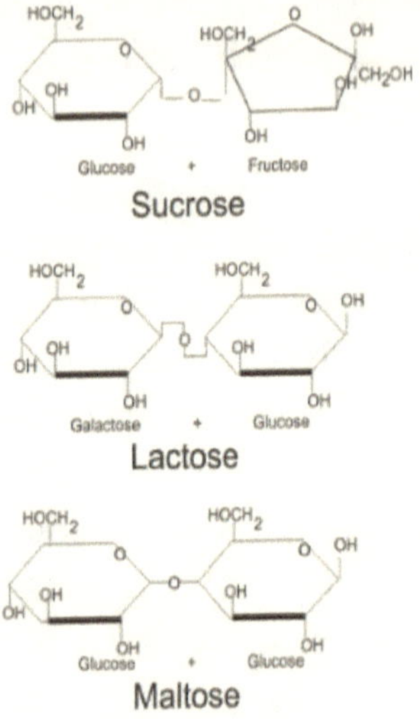

Figure 39: Structure of three common disaccharides.

Carbohydrates also exist in complex forms known as polysaccharides. If these chains of sugar molecules are found in animals, they are referred to as *glycogen*. In plants, they are called *starches*.

For a long time, as exemplified in most text books, carbohydrate metabolism was lumped together in terms of glucose metabolism or glycolysis. Other sugars were rarely mentioned. However, more recent understanding of other sugar metabolism indicated fructose metabolism is very distinct from that of glucose.

Fructose is a monosaccharide found in fruits and vegetables. However, with the introduction of sugar cane, sugar beets and corn sugars, the amount of fructose in the diet has increased exponentially. This is because, as shown in Figure 40, sucrose (cane sugar) is cleaved by the enzyme sucrase into the mono-sugars glucose and fructose before being absorbed into the circulation.

Fructose serves an important survival function. By now, it should be obvious that the humans are designed to survive long periods of food deprivation. The adaptability of our metabolism allows for extended fasts without harm to the individual. We have a natural instinct for sweetness in foods. In addition, fruits are colorful and we are naturally attracted to them. Fruits are abundance in the fall which are important in establishing body fat to sustain us through long winter periods when food sources are scarce.

Upon eating fructose, the sugar is actively transported across the small intestine via the GLUT 5 gut receptor. There is an upregulation of the number of GLUT 5 receptors in the presence of fructose, which allows for greater transport of fructose in subsequent meals. The opposite occurs with starvation.

The important point of distinction between glucose and fructose metabolism resides in the fact that unlike glucose which is utilized in every cell, fructose is metabolized almost exclusively in the liver with little fructose circulating in the blood stream or delivered to peripheral tissues. Fructose is also highly lipogenic, making it ideal for developing the fat mass required to survive winter. In the liver, fructose is metabolized to

VLDL's and then LDL-cholesterol. The fat is subsequently transported via lipoproteins to organs where it is deposited as fat. This is natures mechanism to assure survival during hibernation and long periods of food scarcity.

In nature, fructose is present in the food chain for a short period of time at the end of the growing season. However, in our current environment, the end of the growing season is perpetual. Instead of preparing us for winter, consumption of a fructose-rich diet causes a multitude of clinical problems including insulin resistance, as increase in uric acid, stimulation of lipogenesis resulting in increased levels of triglycerides, cholesterol, and small low-density lipoprotein particles. As we discussed earlier, small low-density lipoprotein particles are correlated with arthrosclerosis. In experiments in rodents, fructose feeding leads to symptoms of metabolic syndrome, including hyperglycemia, hyperinsulinemia as well as obesity, hypertension, and increased levels of triglycerides, fatty acids and cholesterol. The administration of fructose (or sucrose that contains 50% fructose) to humans will cause all features of the metabolic syndrome.

The development of metabolic syndrome seems to be dependent on quantity and duration of fructose consumption. Studies in rats found that a 60% fructose diet causes metabolic syndrome in 10 weeks, whereas a 20% fructose diet extended the development period to 33 weeks. And it took 15 months for a 15% fructose diet to induce insulin resistance.

Studies have shown that fructose increases total cholesterol by elevating LDL cholesterol. Increasing dietary fructose from 3% to 20% of calories increases total cholesterol by 9% and LDL cholesterol by 11%. As little as a 2% increase in dietary fructose raises LDL cholesterol more than 1%. This is direct evidence that in addition to seed oils, fructose contributes to the formation of atherosclerotic plaques. It also points out the difficulty in the interpretation of research data when studies do not control for these variables.

In addition of fructose' indirect effect on atherosclerosis via an increase in total and LDL cholesterol, and small low-density lipoprotein particles, fructose also imparts a direct effect as well. Rats fed a fructose rich diet for two (2) weeks develop endothelial dysfunction. Fructose directly stimulates the endothelial inflammatory processes by upregulating the inflammatory molecule intercellular adhesion molecule-1 (ICAM-1). This suggests that fructose induces inflammatory changes in vascular cells at a concentration achieved in the current American diet.

Fructose can rapidly cause adenosine triphosphate (ATP) depletion in liver cells. Unlike other simple sugars, fructose requires ATP for its metabolism and can cause a rapid ATP depletion. It has been shown that as little as 50 g of fructose (which is slightly more than that present in two 12-oz soft drinks) can induce hepatic ATP depletion in humans when given intravenously. Therefore, consumption of fructose places you at risk for non-alcoholic fatty liver disease (NFALD) and its more severe form, fatty inflammation and scarring.

Currently, the average American is consuming between 70 to 80 grams of fructose per day, which represents between 12 to 15% of their diet. Upwards to 20% of the population exceed 100 grams of fructose per day. And this increase in fructose consumption closely parallels the obesity epidemic which began in the late 1800.

The table (Figure 40) makes it clear that the excess in dietary fructose is primarily from sweeteners, and not necessarily from fruits and vegetables. News about high fructose sweeteners, which have been peppered in the media, only increases the fructose load of 5% compared to sucrose. Whereas, one cup of cane sugar yields 100 grams of fructose because of the cleavage of the bond creating 50% glucose and 50% fructose. Agava nectar, which has been touted as a low glycemic sweetener, is 75% fructose! Even a cup of honey contains 128 grams of fructose. Compare this to blueberries which contains just 3.7 grams of fructose. You would have to eat 35 cups of blueberries to equal one cup of honey!

In conclusion, to reduce the n-6 fatty content of body adipose tissue, these fats need to be metabolized. The diet I am suggesting is one of elimination of all sources of seed oils and fructose (including sucrose or cane sugar). This alone will allow a gradual reduction in body mass. The process can be accelerated by intermittent fasting, and allow 3-4 hours to eat that meal. But the

	Total Sugar (grams)	Sucrose (grams)	Glucose (grams)	Fructose (grams)	Total Fructose
Sugar					
1 c. white sugar	200	200	100	0	100
1c. agave nectar	256	0	72	171	171
1 c. High Fructose 55	235	0	103	129	129
1 c. brown sugar	213	213	106	0	106
1 c. raw honey	279	1	123	140	128
1 c. molasses	252	134	53	58	126
1 c coconut palm sugar	144	114	13	13	70
Fruit					
Apples	13.3	3.3	2.3	7.6	9.3
Banana	15.6	6.5	4.2	2.7	6.0
Blueberries	7.3	0.2	3.5	3.6	3.7
Cantaloupe	8.7	5.4	1.2	1.8	4.5
Cherries	14.6	0.2	8.1	6.2	6.3
Grapefruit	6.2	3.4	1.3	1.2	2.9
Grapes	18.1	0	6.5	7.6	7.6
Lemon	2.5	0.6	1.0	0.8	1.1
Mango	14.8	9.9	0.7	2.9	7.9
Nectarine	8.5	6.2	1.2	6.2	3.1
Orange	9.2	4.2	2.2	4.2	4.6
Papaya	5.9	1.8	1.4	2.7	3.6
Peach	8.7	5.6	1.2	1.3	4.1
Pear	10.5	1.8	1.9	6.4	7.3
Pineapple	11.9	3.1	2.9	2.1	3.7
Plum	7.5	3.0	2.7	1.8	3.3
Raspberries	9.5	2.8	3.5	3.2	4.6
Strawberries	5.8	1.0	2.2	2.5	3.0
Vegetables					
Avocado	0.8	0.1	0.5	0.2	0.3
Beets	6.8	6.5	0.1	0.1	3.3
Carrots	4.7	3.6	0.6	0.6	2.4
Corn	3.2	2.1	0.5	0.5	1.5
Pepper	4.2	0	1.9	2.3	2.3
Sweet Onion	5.0	0.7	2.3	2.0	2.3
Sweet Potato	4.2	2.5	1.0	0.7	1.9
Tomato	2.8	0	1.1	1.4	1.4

intermittent fast must be tailored to suit your needs. You may start by an intermittent fast twice a week. But do not be discouraged. It takes time to reverse the weight gain but weight loss will occur.

Figure 40: Fructose content of common foods. Total fructose is the sum of the monosaccharide (fructose) and the disaccharide (sucrose).

9. Dysbiosis

Humans have evolved alongside the vast numbers of microorganisms that inhabit the body and the gut. In fact, the average human being has as many bacterial cells as his/her own cell numbers! These organisms are mostly populated in the colon, harboring over 100,000,000,000(10^{10}-10^{12}) colony-forming units per gram of feces. It turns out that humans carry between 500-1,000 different bacterial species with the majority belonging in only two distinct phyla: Firmicutes and Bacteroidetes. Other phyla present to a lesser extent include: Actinobacteria, Proteobacteria, Fusobacteria, Spirochaetae and Verrucomicrobia. Only a restricted set of bacterial populations in the nature have been identified in the human body, while approximately 80% of the human bacteria identified by genomic sequencing, are considered uncultivable in the laboratory. Although some prevalent bacterial species in normal individuals are now identified by using whole genome sequencing, more than 60% of species remain unknown.

This complex community of bacteria serves a variety of functions from food digestion, to energy supply, to immune response. While the largest populations are relatively constant between individuals, there is diversity with each individual sheltering over a hundred distinctive species.

Given the symbiotic relationship between these bacteria and intestinal well-being, it should come as little surprise then that factors affecting the gut microbiota, or gut flora, would in turn affect the host. A functioning microbiota is crucial to maintaining a balance of local and systemic homeostasis. A disturbance in the population of microbiota results in gut dysbiosis.

Dysbiosis refers to any imbalance within the gut flora. Numerous studies have shown that an imbalance in dietary PUFAs can lead to dysbiosis. And as you would expect, an individual's omega-6 to omega-3 ratio seen in their adipose tissue profile is reflected in changes in the microbiota. Studies have shown that animals with high tissue n-3 levels are associated with anti-inflamma-tory gut bacteria, while high n-6 levels are associated with pro-inflammatory bacteria. Studies conducted in mice have found that diets rich in safflower oil (omega-6) reduces the abundance of *Bacteroidetes*, while enrich-ing the populations of *Firmicutes, Actinobacteria and Pro-teobacteria*. In addition, safflower oil stimulated the growth of δ-*Proteobacteria* by enhancing bacterial genes, giving them a competitive advantage over other bacte-rial groups that colonize the GI tract.

Mice fed a diet rich in omega-6 PUFAs (corn oil) results in bacterial overgrowth and dysbiosis. The high n-6 PUFA diet, is associated with bacterial invasion of the intestinal epithelial cell layer. Corn oil supplementa-tion causes hyperinsulinemia.

Inflammation is the result of the secretion of lip-opolysaccharide (LPS) from gram negative bacteria. LPS is the major component of the outer membrane of the bacteria, and when released, is considered an endotoxin due to its potent stimulatory effect on the immune sys-tem. The pro-inflammatory bacteria, commonly found in animals consuming a high omega-6 diet, produce greater amounts of LPS while the bacterium of high omega-3 fed animals do not produce nearly as much LPS, and thus have less inflammatory significance.

Figure 41 shows the correlation of tissue PUFA with components of the microbiota from animal experi-ments. Chronic systemic exposure from LPS due to dysbiosis leads to a disorder called Metabolic Endotox-emia (ME). Metabolic Endotoxemia is characterized by increased plasma concentrations of LPS with chronic inflammation, and is linked to diabetes, obesity, dyslipidemia, neurological and cardiovascular disease. Animals studies have consistently correlated high tissue omega-6 levels with dysbiosis, ME, and a higher incidence rate of chronic diseases.

LPS Producing/Pro-Inflammatory Bacteria (High Omega-6)	LPS Suppressing/Anti-Inflammatory Bacteria (High Omega-3)
Phylum *Proteobacteria* and its members	*Bifidobacterium*
- *Enterobacteriaceae*,	
- *Escherichia coli*	
- *Gamma proteobacteria*	
- *Delta proteobacteria*	
Genus *Prevotella*	*Akkermansia muciniphila*
Genus *Fusobacterium*	*Lactobacillus*
Clostridium cluster XI	*Clostridium* clusters IV and XIVa
Segmented filamentous bacteria (*Candidatus savagella*)	*Enterococcus faecium*
	Bacteroidetes

Figure 41: Lipopolysaccharide producing bacteria observed in animals with varying PUFA ratios.

Chronic low-grade inflammation, as we saw in previous chapters, is characterized by elevated circulating levels of inflammatory cytokines, such as tumor necrosis factor-alpha (TNF-α), interleukin (IL)-1, and IL-6. A primary cause of chronic low-grade inflammation is metabolic endotoxemia. LPS binds to Toll-like receptor-4 (TLR4) which activates inflammasomes leading to increased cytokine production and an inflammatory cascade.

Diet is known to be an important modulating factor of metabolic endotoxemia and chronic low-grade inflammation. Mice fed a diet high in omega-6 fatty acids exhibit higher levels of metabolic endotoxemia and systemic low-grade inflammation, while omega-3 fatty acids dramatically reduces endotoxemia and inflammatory symptoms. Ghosh (*et al.*,2012) observed that feeding high-fat diets rich in n-6 PUFA promotes bacterial overgrowth but depletes microbes from the Bacteroidetes and Firmicutes phyla. This change in the microbiota corresponded with increased body mass, with infiltration of macrophages and neutrophils. Fish oil supplementation restored the microbiota, reduced the inflammatory cell infiltration, and promoted regulatory T-cell recruitment. However, fish oil supplementation was associated with increased oxidative stress, evident by the increased presence of 4-hydroxynonenal, a product of lipid peroxidation.

Interestingly, these effects are eliminated by antibiotic therapy thereby suggesting direct involvement by the gut microbiota. Elevated tissue omega-3 fatty acids enhance secretion of intestinal alkaline phosphatase (IAP), which induces changes in the gut bacteria population resulting in decreased lipopolysaccharide production.

Inflammatory Bowel Diseases

Given the higher concentrations of LPS in the gut as a result from dysbiosis, one would expect to see a cause and effect relationship with elevated populations of gram negative bacteria and the integrity of the mucosal epithelium of the gut. In fact, Omega-6 PUFAs have been shown in rodent studies to exacerbate Inflammatory Bowel Disease through dysbiosis, representing a 30% increased risk.

Feeding mice 20% corn oil for 5 weeks significantly reduces *Bacteroides* species in the gut, while increasing intestinal epithelial cell death. In addition, these mice have high levels of bacteria from the Clostridium and Enterobacteriaceae phyla, which are associated with inflammatory bowel disease. In contrast, mice fed corn oil diets supplemented with fish oil have enriched beneficial microbes (*Lactobacillus*) and lower levels of *Enterobacteriaceae* and *Clostridia* species. Fish oil also reduces neutrophil infiltration as well. Canola oil, which contains n-3, n-6 PUFAs and oleic acid (monounsaturated), alters the microbiota similar to corn oil.

Colorectal Cancer

Several recent studies have looked at the composition of the gut microbiome associated with patients with colorectal cancer. In each of these studies, there was a significant shift in the composition of the gut microbiome in patients with cancer as compared to that in healthy controls. Colorectal patients are shown to have increased levels of certain bacterial species such as *Bacteroides fragilis, Enterococcus, Escherichia/Shigella, Klebsiella, Streptococcus, Peptostreptococcus, Roseburia* and decreased abundance in butyrate-producing *Lachnospiraceae*.

This colorectal cancer-associated dysbiosis, is

observed in both the microbiome taken from feces, as well as the mucosa-associated microbiome from tumor biopsy specimens. These studies clearly show an association between abnormalities in the gut microbiome and colorectal cancer. Zackular (*et al.*, 2013) further demonstrated that changes in the gut microbiome associated with inflammation and tumorigenesis directly contributes to tumorigenesis, and suggested that interventions affecting the composition of the microbiome may be a strategy to prevent the development of colon cancer.

Recent studies have also demonstrated that n-3 fatty acids from fish oil could prevent colon cancer development. Evidences show that n-3 PUFAs act at different stages of cancer development, limiting tumor cell proliferation, increase apoptotic potential, promoting cell differentiation and possibly limit angiogenesis. In fact, a study from Japan suggests **omega-3 polyunsaturated fatty acids could reduce the risk of colorectal cancer by 74 percent!**

Gut bacteria are not only strongly related to gastrointestinal cancer but also prostate cancer. The systemic inflammation caused by pathogenic gut bacteria plays a pivotal role in development of prostate cancer. Poutahidis *et al.* found mice infected with the bacteria *Helicobacter hepaticus* had significantly increased incidence of prostate neoplasia and micro invasive adenocarcinoma lesions of the prostate.

Intestinal Dysbiosis in Systemic Diseases

As we observed in previous chapters, there is a

triad of interlinked diseases, and we see this again in intestinal dysbiosis. In addition to local gastrointestinal diseases, dysbiosis is also associated with systemic diseases such as obesity, diabetes, and atherosclerosis. There are many metabolic diseases associated with chronic inflammation induced by lipopolysaccharide, as well as other bacterial metabolites.

Atherosclerosis

There is significant evidence that the gut microbiota is involved in the development of atherosclerosis, and to support this claim are numerous studies that implicate microbial byproducts in atherogenesis. Specific bacterial DNA has been identified in atherosclerotic plaques which are linked to bacteria found in oral or gut samples from patients with atherosclerosis. DNA sequencing of fecal samples has found the *Bacteroides* were diminished and *Ruminococcus* overgrown in atherosclerotic patients.

LPS, as discussed earlier, is released from gram-negative bacteria which then leads to a chronic inflammatory state that accelerates atherosclerosis in humans and rodents. For example, delivery of C. *pneumoniae* to the vessel wall of carotid arteries in mice increases the development of atherosclerosis. Repeated intravenous and intraperitoneal administration of LPS accelerates atherosclerosis in rabbits and mice.

In addition to lipopolysaccharides, certain bacterial metabolites can exert cytotoxicity and promote inflammation, tissue injury, and have been linked to atherosclerosis. Trimethylamine N-oxide (TMAO) has been shown to contribute to the development and progression of atherosclerosis and cardiovascular disease. In 2013, Tang *et al*. published an article in the New England Journal of Medicine demonstrating the critical role of dietary choline and gut microbiota in TMAO production. The authors measured plasma and urinary levels of TMAO and plasma choline in healthy participants before and after the suppression of intestinal microbiota with oral broad-spectrum antibiotics. They also examined the relationship between fasting plasma levels of TMAO and incident major adverse cardiovascular events (death, myocardial infarction, or stroke) during three years of follow-up in 4,007 patients undergoing elective coronary angiography. They found plasma levels of TMAO were markedly suppressed after the administration of antibiotics and then reappeared after withdrawal of antibiotics. Increased plasma levels of TMAO were associated with an increased risk of a major adverse cardiovascular events.

p-cresyl sulfate, is another bacterial metabolite which has been shown to readily penetrate the endothelial cell membrane and cause endothelial damage. p-cresyl sulfate induces the shedding of the endothelial microparticles we discussed earlier. Elevated plasma levels of p-cresyl sulfate are associated with the high concentrations of endothelial microparticles. These microparticles are related to increased arterial stiffness and act as pro-thrombotic and pro-inflammatory mediators. The role of p-cresyl sulfate in mediating the release of the endothelial microparticles was confirmed by *in vitro* studies using cultured human endothelial cells.

There is a correlation with elevated *p*-cresyl sulfate in plasma and the risk of cardiovascular disease. It is believed that *p*-cresyl may accumulate in vascular endothelial and smooth muscle cells, and induce oxidative stress through the production of radical oxygen species (ROS), thereby resulting in the development of cytotoxicity.

The other widely studied toxin generated by the gut microbiota is indoxyl sulfate. Indoxyl sulfate is a by-product of the intestinal microbial flora and has been shown to promote the progression of renal and cardiovascular disease by inducing oxidative stress, inflammation and fibrosis.

Earlier, we discussed the role of cholesterol in the development and progression of coronary artery disease. Three Lactobacillus strains are known to assimilated cholesterol directly from the gut. Consumption of commercially available probiotic products which contains *Lactobacillus plantarum* results in decreased circulating leptin levels, smaller myocardial infarcts, and greater recovery from heart attack.

Obesity

In studies conducted on mice, the microbiome of obese mice have higher levels of firmicutes and lower levels of *bacteroides*, similar to what we see with high omega 6 intake. In normal mice, the opposite is true. Interestingly, transplanting the gut bacteria from obese mice to normal mice causes the normal mice to gain weight.

Obese children have a microbiota enriched with *Enterobacteriaceae* and reduced *Bacteroides*. Carbohydrate-restricted diets reverse this trend and increases Bacteroidetes and decreased Firmicutes.

Mice who receive a gut bacteria transplant from obese donors develop an increase in body mass as well as an increase in adipose tissue compared to those receiving transplants from lean donors. Co-housing lean and obese mice prevents the increase in adiposity in obese cage mates. What is interesting is the co-habitation transformed their microbiota to a lean-like state!

However, the microbial protection from increased adiposity was only possible with a suitable host diet. Besides probiotics, other gut bacteria could also protect humans from obesity. *Bacteroidetes* phylum, *particularly Bacteroides spp.*, is suggested to be mainly responsible for protection against increased adiposity.

Diabetes

Changes in the gut bacteria contribute to diabetes. LPS is believed to be a causative factor in triggering the onset of diet-induced type-2 diabetes. Murri et al. found the number of *Clostridium, Bacteroides and Veillonella* significantly increased, and the number of *Lactobacillus, Bifidobacterium, Blautia coccoides/Eubacterium* rectale group and *Prevotella* significantly decreased in children with type-1 diabetes. Meanwhile, *Bifidobacterium spp.* had a significantly positive correlation with improved glucose tolerance, glucose-induced insulin secretion and normalized inflammatory tone with high-fat prebiotic treated mice.

Bifidobacterium treatment improves the inflammatory and metabolic status in mice. Glucose intolerance is moderately blunted, and insulin sensitivity and fasting hyperinsulinemia are completely normalized. In addition, antibiotic therapy has a positive result in animal diabetic models.

A paper published in Nature (2014) makes the observation that artificial sweeteners (aspartame, sucralose, and saccharin) causes blood glucose abnormalities in mice and some humans. The changes in glucose tolerance appear to be driven by changes to the microbiome. The investigators gave mice one of these three sweeteners in their water. They found they all three sweeteners induced a blood sugar disturbance even compared to mice who drank sugary water!

The investigators hypothesized that gut microbes are responsible for the results. And to prove this hypothesis, they gave antibiotics to the mice: One group received ciprofloxacin and metronidazole, a broad-spectrum approach focusing on gram-negative bacteria, and another group received vancomycin, aimed against gram-positive bacteria. Both treatments, when given for four weeks, eliminated the differences in glucose tolerance between sweetener-fed mice and controls.

The glucose intolerance could also be triggered by a microbial transplant. Microbes from mice who had been drinking saccharin were transplanted via feces into germ-free mice which caused the recipients to show an impaired glucose tolerance; whereas microbes from mice who had been drinking glucose did not.

This effect of artificial sweeteners seems to hold true for humans as well. In an experiment involving 381 nondiabetic participants, long-term consumption of artificial sweeteners was associated with measures of obesity and glucose intolerance.

Saccharin increases numbers of Bacteroides bacteria in the gut as well as increases the density of bacteria in the Enterobacteriaceae group while decreasing the number of certain beneficial bacteria, such as *Akkermansia mucinophila*.

Maintaining a Healthy Microbiota

Besides dietary supplementation with a probiotic, elimination of omega-6 PUFAs from the diet will eliminate pro-inflammatory bacteria from the gut. Omega-3 PUFAs (EPA and DHA) can reversed bacterial overgrowth and reduced inflammation by recruiting regulatory T-cells to the small intestine. However, there is not a similar protection by saturated fatty acids. Dietary fish oil strengthened intestinal barrier function and reduced plasma endotoxin levels in swine.

A recent study showed that mice fed fish oil had

decreased abundance of *Helicobacter* and *Pseudomonas* and Firmicutes, organisms associated with ulcers, infection, and weight gain. One mechanism that may account for dietary n-3 PUFA's reduction of *Helicobacter* and *Pseudomonas* is that those organisms are sensitive to the direct bactericidal effects of EPA and DHA. Bacterial killing by n-3 PUFAs and other fatty acids is likely important to the overall composition of the microbiota and the function of the intestinal barrier.

10. Neurological Implications

The brain contains high levels of polyunsaturated fatty acids and is therefore highly sensitive to oxidative stress. The brain consumes about 20–30% of inspired oxygen, making it an ideal target of free radical attack.

Fatty acids and lipids are major components in brain structure, found principally in two structural components: The neuronal membrane and in myelin sheaths. Myelin is a fatty white substance that surrounds the axon of some nerve cells, and serves to increase the speed at which impulses propagate along the nerve fiber. The integrity of the myelin is extremely importance for the proper functions of axons in the nervous system. Any damage to the myelin can lead to major neurological dysfunctions. This is important as we explore the effects of PUFAs on various diseases involving myelin dysfunction.

There are many studies that emphasize the major role dietary omega-3 fatty acids have on the normal functions of myelin. If omega-3 fatty acids are not available in the diet, amyelination, dysmyelination or demyelination may occur. The turnover rate of myelin is also very slow during aging, and therefore affects the rate of repair to damaged sections of myelin.

The principal omega-3 PUFA in the central nervous system is docosahexaenoic acid (DHA), representing 10–20% of the total fatty acid composition. The protein component in the brain is stable, whereas the lipid component has a relatively high turnover rate.

Omega–3 deficiency results in a significant decrease in the neuron size in many brain areas. In addition, omega–3 deficiency induces a significant reduction in catecholamine levels, in glucose utilization, and in brain phospholipid synthesis.

We now know, PUFAs have been linked to several diseases in neurology and psychiatry, including depression, bipolar disorder, schizophrenia, attention-deficit–hyperactive disorder and neurodegenerative diseases, such as Alzheimer's disease, Parkinson's disease, Huntington's disease, and ALS.

Spinal Cord injury

The opposing effects of omega-3 versus omega-6 fatty acids can be seen in models of spinal cord injury. Lang-Lazdunski *et al.* noted that the administration of omega-3 fatty acid within the first hour in a rat model of spinal cord injury, led to a decrease in nerve loss, and an improved functional outcome. In a similar model of hemi section of the cord in adult rats, DHA (as well as the precursor acid, LNA) induced significant neuroprotection. These omega-3 PUFAs reduced nerve cell loss, oligodendrocyte loss, and decreased nerve cell death following injury. This correlates with a significantly improved functional outcome. In rat hemi section and compression spinal cord injury, long-chain omega-3 PUFAs (such as docosahexaenoic acid), administered within the first hour after injury, can reduce neuronal and glial cell death, limit oxidative stress and the inflammatory cascade triggered by the primary injury, thereby improving neurological function. By contrast, when animals received an omega-6 fatty acid (arachidonic acid (AA)) following injury, there was an exacerbation of the injury, and the initial lesion was seen to spread, with formation of secondary lesions and worsened functional outcome.

There are many additional studies that support the observation that PDUFAs can modify spinal cord injury. In a model of spinal cord injury induced by compression, DHA injected intravenously within the first hour after injury induced significant neuroprotection. Furthermore, in a subset of animals who had received the DHA bolus and were also exposed to a DHA-enriched diet, performed significantly better than the DHA-bolus only group. DHA decreased lipid peroxidation, protein oxidation and also the oxidation of nucleic acids.

A favorable outcome from a spinal cord injury is dependent on protection on myelinated axons. If even a small number of axons were spared (10-15%), the outcome would be significantly improved due to the plasticity of the nervous system. So, it is clearly important to examine the effect of omega-3 fatty acids on injured axons. As it turns out, following spinal cord injury, DHA induces a significant protection of myelin. These observations suggest that the acute administration of long-chain omega-3 PUFAs, within a realistic time window after SCI, could confer significant neuroprotection.

Brain Edema

Brain edema occurs when water content of brain tissue is increased. Severe brain injury leads to brain edema which is usually irreversible and leads to marked increase in intracranial pressure and death due to the expansion of the brain against the skull. The edema is initiated by the release of free-radicals which disrupt the microvascular network. And once initiated, free radical injury is a self-perpetuating process with increasing damage, generating more free radicals

Polyunsaturated fatty acids (PUFAs), arachidonic acid in particular, are well known, potent inducers of edema in the brain, while monounsaturated and saturated long chain fatty acids do not. Polyunsaturated fatty acids (including arachidonic, linoleic, linolenic, and docosahexaenoic acids) induces edema in slices of rat brain cortex. This cellular edema was specific to polyunsaturated fatty acids, since neither saturated fatty acids nor mono-saturated fatty acid containing a single double bond had such effect.

Intracerebral injection of polyunsaturated fatty acids PUFAs, (including linolenic acid (18:3) and arachidonic acid (20:4)), causes a significant increase in cerebral water and sodium content in the brain, with gross as well as microscopic evidence of edema. Again, as in previous experiments, saturated fatty acids and mono-unsaturated fatty acid are not effective in inducing brain edema. There is a major decrease in brain potassium content concurrent with the edema as well. In addition, the induction of brain edema by arachidonic acid is dose dependent and maximal between 24 and 48 hours after perfusion. These data indicate that arachidonic acid and other PUFAs have the ability to induce brain edema, and initiate the development of brain edema in various disease states.

The involvement of superoxide free radicals and lipid peroxidation in brain swelling induced by free fatty acids has been studied in brain slices as well. The polyunsaturated fatty acids linoleic acid (18:2), linolenic acid (18:3), arachidonic acid (20:4), and docosahexaenoic acid (22:6) causes brain swelling concomitant with increases in superoxide and membrane lipid peroxidation. Palmitic acid (16:0) and oleic acid (18:1) have no such effect. These in vitro data support the hypothesis that both superoxide radicals and lipid peroxidation are involved in the mechanism of polyunsaturated fatty acid-induced brain edema.

However, the concentration of arachidonic acid required to induce swelling is about 20 times higher than the concentration required to induce inhibition of mitochondrial respiratory function (Hillered and Chan, 1988). The reversal of brain swelling occurs without recovery of mitochondrial respiratory function, suggesting that swelling is a secondary importance to that of brain mitochondrial dysfunction.

The effects of omega-6 fatty acids have a direct implication for stroke victims. Arachidonic acid or docosahexaenoic acid, administrated after 60 minutes in a rat model of brain injury, clearly aggravate the cerebral ischemic injury. The aggravation is manifested as enlargement of areas of cerebral infarction and increased impairment of motor activity, in a concentration dependent manner.

The augmentation of injury in AA and DHA treatment animals is accompanied by increases in the permeability of the blood-brain barrier, brain edema, inflammatory cell infiltration, and malondialdehyde (MDA) production. It is hypothesized that malondialdehyde has a significant role in inducing edema in traumatic brain injury patients. Furthermore, either AA or DHA alone increases the hydrogen peroxide-induced oxidative burden. Taken together, these findings demonstrate the detrimental effect of omega-6 PUFA on the progression of brain injury.

Alzheimer's disease

Alzheimer's disease is the most common form of dementia in the elderly, characterized by degeneration in selective brain regions involved in memory and emotional behaviors. Alzheimer's disease is a progressive disease which gradually reduces the ability to learn, think, and memorize, ultimately robbing the patient with his/her memory. The histological hallmarks of the disease are deposition of plaques and intracellular neurofibrillary tangles (NFTs) around neurons of the brain. The beta-amyloid plaques are clumps of protein deposits and cellular material that form outside and around neurons. The neurofibrillary tangles are fibers composed mostly of the protein tau that build up inside nerve cells.

Alzheimer's disease is defined in three stages: mild cognitive impairment, early-stage Alzheimer disease, and late-stage Alzheimer disease. Patients are usually diagnosed on the basis of the severity of symptoms.

There is increasing evidence that supports a role for oxidative damage to lipids, protein and nucleic acids in the pathogenesis of Alzheimer's disease. Numerous studies show an increase in DNA, RNA, and protein oxidation in regions of brain from late stage Alzheimer's disease patients compared to normal control subjects. In addition, markers of oxidative damage are elevated in subjects with mild cognitive impairment. It is interesting to note that the oxidative damage seen early in the disease are similar to those observed in late stage disease suggesting oxidative damage is an early event in the pathogenesis.

As we learned in previous chapters, Lipid peroxidation is the major sources of free radical-mediated injury that directly damages nerve membranes and mitochondria; as well as creating a number of secondary products. These aldehydes, (including malondialdehyde (MDA), 4-hydroxy-2-nonenal (HNE)), and acrolein, are responsible of extensive cellular damage in the nervous system. In addition to aldehyde formation, peroxidation of PUFAs produce fatty acid esters: ispoprostanes and neuroprostanes. Neuroprostanes are produced by peroxidation of docosahexaenoic acid (DHA).

Several studies indicate that levels of acrolein and HNE are elevated in late-stage Alzheimer's disease. More recently, additional studies show a significant elevation of 4-hydroxyhexenal (HHE), in vulnerable regions the Alzheimer's brain. Although HHE has only recently been the focus in Alzheimer's disease, this finding is of particular significance since it is the by-product of peroxidation of omega-3 PUFAs including docosahexaenoic acid (DHA), the predominant PUFA in the brain. Concentrations of DHA in the brain are 30 – 50 times those of arachidonic acid, the predominate omega-6 PUFA, suggesting that oxidative stress of brain tissue is the source of HHE.

The beta-amyloid plaques, the hallmark of Alzheimer's disease, is positive for HNE. The modification of the beta-amyloid may contribute to the toxicity associated with the amyloid deposits. In addition, HNE is found in neurofibrillary tangles the other histological marker for the disease. HNE at low concentrations has been shown to impair glucose transport, is implicated in mitochondrial dysfunction in neurons of AD patients.

Mitochondrial dysfunction is another feature of Alzheimer's disease (Castellani *et al.*, 2002). Defects in the mitochondria are the same defects of the electron transport chain we discussed earlier. It has been shown that oxidative species (ROS), through mitochondrial dysfunction, leads to neuron and synapse loss (Melov *et al.*, 2007). This Mitochondrial dysfunction and oxidative damage have been investigated in the transgenic mouse model. These mice exhibited increased oxidative stress, manifested by increased hydrogen peroxide production and lipid peroxidation (Yao *et al.*, 2009; Reddy, 2011).

Multiple Sclerosis

Multiple sclerosis is a chronic inflammatory disease of the central nervous system, associated with demyelination and neurodegeneration. Although the exact case is unknown, multiple sclerosis is considered to be an autoimmune disease. Risk factors for the disease include being between 15-60 years of age, and women have about two to three times the risk for multiple sclerosis than men. Multiple sclerosis symptoms and signs depend on where the nerves are demyelinated and may include:

- visual changes including double vision or loss of vision
- numbness
- tingling or weakness (weakness may range from mild to severe)
- paralysis
- vertigo or dizziness
- erectile dysfunction (ED, impotence)
- pregnancy problems
- incontinence (or conversely, urinary retention)
- muscle spasticity
- incoordination of muscles
- tremor
- painful involuntary muscle contractions
- slurred speech
- fatigue.

The mechanisms of tissue injury are poorly understood, but recent data suggest that mitochondrial injury may play an important role in this process. As with Alzheimer's disease, oxidized lipids are present in active multiple sclerosis plaques. Similarly, lipid peroxidation-derived structures (malondialdehyde and oxidized phospholipids) are seen in the cytoplasm of oligodendrocytes and some astrocytes of the brain. The extent of lipid and DNA oxidation correlates significantly with inflammation, determined by the number of macrophages in the lesions. This strongly suggests oxidative injury of neurons are associated with active demyelination and axonal or neuronal injury in multiple sclerosis.

Low density lipoprotein (LDL), which as we discussed at length, is the major carrier of plasma cholesterol. As with cardiovascular disease, oxy-LDL may enter the neurons of early multiple sclerosis (MS) lesions as a result of blood-brain barrier damage. MDA-LDL (Malondialdehyde) and 4-HNE-LDL (4-hydroxynonenal) are present in the foamy macrophages in actively demyelinating MS plaques suggesting that a large proportion of the plasma LDL which enters the neurons of MS plaques is oxidized. Lipid peroxidation and oxidized LDL uptake by activated macrophages in the early stages of MS plaque development may play important roles in demyelination similar to the processes in arthrosclerosis plaques!

Amyotrophic lateral sclerosis

Amyotrophic lateral sclerosis (ALS), is a disorder characterized by the slow death of motor neurons. In ALS, the sensory neurons are spared, only affecting neurons that control voluntary muscles. ALS is characterized by stiff muscles, muscle twitching, and gradually worsening weakness resulting in difficulty speaking, swallowing, moving, and eventually breathing. Most people with ALS die from respiratory failure, usually within three to five years from the onset of symptoms.

While the pathophysiology of the disease is unknown, the defining feature of ALS is the death of both upper and lower motor neurons in the motor cortex of the brain, the brain stem, and the spinal cord. Prior to their destruction, motor neurons develop protein-rich inclusions in their cell bodies and axons.

ALS occurs both sporadically (sALS) in 90% of patients, and as a familial disorder (fALS) (involving family mutations), in about 10% of patients. fALS is caused by a dominant inherited mutations in the super-oxide dismutase (SOD) gene which encodes for super-oxide dismutase. SOD is an enzyme found in all cells that catalyzes the breakdown of the superoxide radical into either ordinary molecular oxygen (O_2) or hydrogen peroxide (H_2O_2). fALS cases are indistinguishable from sALS, suggesting that the SOD1-mutant animal model provides insight into similar and converging pathogenic mechanisms shared by both sporadic and familial forms. Over 100 SOD1 mutations have been identified in fALS patients.

The mechanism of sALS caused by mutant SOD1 (mSOD1) is not known. Many hypotheses have been proposed to explain the toxicity of ALS mutant SOD1 proteins. One hypothesis suggests that mSOD1 become misfolded and consequently form intracellular plaques which interfere with essential proteins for normal cellu-lar function. Another hypothesis proposes the oxidative damage is caused by enhanced oxidative stress.

Elevated levels of reactive free radicals (ROS) and the formation of insoluble protein complexes of mu-tant SOD1 protein have been detected in spinal cords of transgenic mice prior to motor neuron degeneration It may be that these two phenomena are linked, Oxidative damage hypothesis is further supported by considerable evidence of increased ROS-mediated oxidative stress, such as malondialdehyde, 4-hydroxyl-2-nonenal (HNE), oxidized proteins, DNA, and membrane phospholipids, in sporadic and fALS.

An examination of 31 patients suffering from ALS shows elevated levels of malondialdehyde (MDA) and HNE in their plasma as well as spinal fluid when compared to healthy individuals. The HNE levels were positively correlated with extent of disease but not rate of progression.

If one examines the spinal cord and ventral horn motor neurons of ALS patients, you will find an increase in HNE levels, as well as an increase in HNE-modified proteins, indicating that HNE plays a critical role motor neuron degeneration in ALS. If you compare those proteins that are modified by HNE, you find an increase in the amount of HNE significantly bound to dihydropyrimidinase related protein 2 (DRP-2), and to the heat-shock protein 70 (HSP70). DRP-2 is involved in axonal outgrowth and modulation of extracellular signals. Interestingly, DRP-2 is found in the neurofibrillary tangles of Alzheimer's disease.

Members of the Hsp70 family are very strongly upregulated by heat stress, hence the term heat shock proteins. Heat Shock Proteins exist in virtually all living organisms. The Hsp70s are an important part of the cell's machinery for protein folding, and help to protect cells from stress. Therefore, Hsp70 chaperone activity could play a crucial role in the pathophysiology of motor neurons disease, in particular in the context of mutations of SOD1. The Hsp70 is a chaperone protein that helps newly synthesized proteins to be folded and transported across the nerve membrane. In addition, Hsp70 can act to protect proteins from oxidative stress by stabilizing them and thereby preventing the partial unfolding and possible aggregation which would occur without Hsp70.

Thirty-one (31) patients suffering from ALS, were compared to twenty-four (24) patients suffering from Parkinson's disease, and 30 healthy subjects. Plasma levels of lipid peroxidation (malondialdehyde), and the activity of antioxidant enzymes (SOD), were measured. MDA is significantly different in both neurodegenerative diseases versus control population. A trend for an increase of oxidized glutathione was noted in ALS patients. A further analysis showed that SOD activity was significantly decreased in ALS.

While protein misfolding seems to be at the root cause of ALS, it is clear that these patients cannot compensate for the free radical formation due to changes SOD as shown by the elevated lipid oxidation products. While direct studies have not been conducted with omega-6 fatty acids in this patient population, it would be prudent nonetheless to avoid polyunsaturated fats that form oxidation products such as MDA and HNE.

11. Lipofuscin and Aging

Lipofuscin

One of the most notable changes that occur in mammalian cells with aging is the gradual accumulation of cellular inclusions known as <u>lipofuscin</u> or age pigments. These pigments were observed as early as 1842, making them one of the oldest, if not the most widely recognized, change which takes place in all cells with increasing age.

McGraw-Hill Concise Dictionary of Modern Medicine defines Lipofuscin as *brown pigment granules representing lipid-containing residues of lysosome digestion*

*and considered one of the aging or "wear and tear" pigments;
found in liver, kidney, heart muscle, adrenal, and ganglion
cells.* In other words, lipofuscin, is an age pigment; a
dark pigment seen with increasing frequency with advancing age in the cytoplasm of cells. A simple analogy
is "cellular garbage".

Durand G. Desnoyers noted that the lipofuscin
bodies observed in nerve cell sections, and the quantity
of those pigments in neurons, were correlated to the age
of the individual. Microscopic studies have shown the
presence of this pigments in the cells of most tissues in
vertebrates as well as invertebrates. The comparable
morphology, composition and physicochemical properties of these various pigments suggests that they are all
produced by the same biochemical mechanism.

Many references still label this pigment as "age-
related". Yet back in 1967, Hartroft and Porta published
in *Present Knowledge in Nutrition,* their observation that
the "age pigment," (lipofuscin), was formed in proportion to the amount of polyunsaturated fat and oxidants
in the diet. The rate of pigment formation is increased
by vitamin E deficiency, and by increased intake of polyunsaturated fatty acids. In addition, the rate of
lipofuscin formation can be experimentally manipulated. Exposure of 40% oxygen to cells in cell culture in
order to create oxidative stress, promotes lipofuscin accumulation, whereas 8% oxygen and treatment with antioxidants diminishes it. Therefore, we can surmise that
lipid peroxidation reactions are implicated in lipofuscin

formation.

Unfortunately, lipofuscin inclusions are not degraded, and cannot be removed from the cell via traditional pathways (via exocytosis). Therefore, lipofuscin accumulation in cells is inevitable, especially in cells that do not divide or divide infrequently (i.e. nerve and cardiac cells). But we can control the rate at which these inclusions are deposited.

What we now know is lipofuscin is produced by:

- the peroxidation of the polyunsaturated fatty acids of cellular membranes by free radicals;

- the reaction of lipid peroxidation end-products(s) with proteins (i.e. malondialdehyde, 4-Hydroxynonenal, etc.),

- the combination of those polymerized elements and peroxidized lipids.

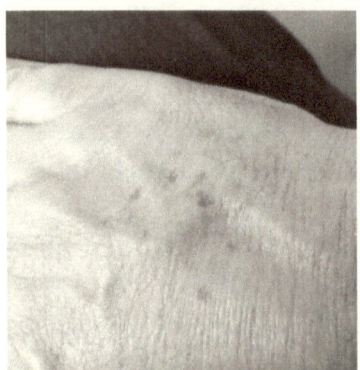

In other words, age related pigments are the result of the peroxidation of the unstable double bonds found in polyunsaturated fats.

From an evolutionary perspective, cellular damage from free radicals, has been present since the beginning of

Figure 42: Lipofuscin (liver or age spots). Spots arise as a result of lipofuscin-containing cells.

life. With the evolution of more complex cells, there necessitated a development of defenses against these *damaging* reactions, as well as the removal and replacement of altered parts, including those no longer needed by the cells. Antioxidants such as vitamin E, superoxide dismutase, glutathione peroxidase, and peroxidase work well in keeping the peroxidation of unsaturated fats in check. While these defenses work, flooding the cellular apparatus with large qualities of unsaturated fats, which were not present during the evolution of the defenses, overloads the cell resulting in lipofuscin formation.

The relationship of lipofuscin to dietary polyunsaturated fats has been fairly well established. Mann and Yates have measured the lipofuscin and melanin contents of nerve cells in eighteen (18) subjects; nine (9) of British Nationality, and nine (9) from Sri Lanka, with both groups being matched for age and sex. Lipofuscin content was increased by age in the British cases, suggesting that this change in composition may be related to differences in diet, particularly in respect of the amount of polyunsaturated fat consumed by the two populations. The Sri Lankan cuisine is mostly rice, served with fish, chicken, beef, mutton, or goat.

The presence of lipofuscin granules has been implicated in a number of disease states. However, we cannot say for certain whether the disease is a direct consequence of the pigments, or whether the pigments are simply a marker of lipid peroxidation. Terman and

Brunk noted that myocardial aging includes an accumulation of lipofuscin. These changes are caused by continuous oxidative stress with advancing age; because the cellular turnover machinery is inherently imperfect, as well as an over exposure of the tissue to polyunsaturated fats. Because lipofuscin-laden lysosomes fail to degrade the pigment, the cells are in short supply of lysosomal enzymes. This lysosomal damage eventually results in functional failure and death of cardiac muscle cells.

Examination of cardiac cells from necropsies and biopsy specimens has revealed evidence that the mitochondria themselves can be transformed into granules of lipofuscin. These granules have been shown to arise from the peroxidative destruction of polyunsaturated fats in lipid membranes. In fact, the occurrence of brown atrophy of the heart in relatively young persons is indicative of an elevated rate of lipofuscin formation. Peroxidative damage to the myocardium is unfortunately, cumulative and irreversible.

The central nervous system, including the eye and brain is DHA-rich. And, as expected, lipofuscin is present in virtually every type of neuron, but is

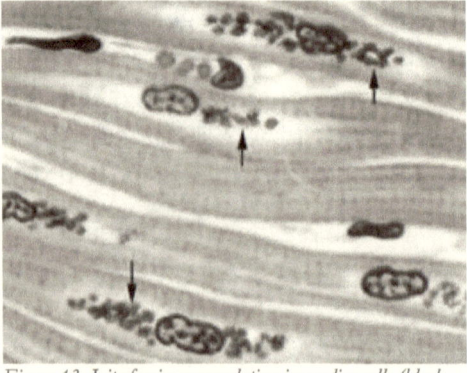

Figure 43: Lipofuscin accumulation in cardiac cells (black arrows).

most abundant in the largest neurons. The age-dependent accumulation of lipofuscin in brain cells is one of the most consistent features of aging. While lipofuscin granules are detectable neurons in the brains of young children, the levels are minimal. Neuron in the brains of young children have small amounts of lipofuscin granules, but become progressively and markedly more abundant between the second and ninth decade of life.

We should expect that lipid peroxidation may contribute to some degenerative brain disorders, in addition to vision-threatening macular pathologies. There is a family of at least eight rare, and genetically distinct, neurodegenerative diseases associated with accumulation of lipofuscin in cells known as <u>neuronal ceroid lipofuscinoses</u> (NCL); also known as Batten disease. The NCL diseases are associated with variable, yet progressive symptoms including seizures, dementia, visual loss, and/or cerebral atrophy. Patients with NCL have shortened life expectancy, with life span depending on the type of NCL that a patient has. Life expectancy ranges from age six (6) years to early teens. Onset is usually between ages four (4) and ten (10) years for CLN3 disease, classic juvenile.

If the accumulation of lipofuscin within neurons is involved in their age-related demise, it is tempting to ascribe a role for this substance in cognitive decline. Alzheimer's Disease, another of the diseases of aging, may be due to increasing lipofuscin content in neuronal cells. It has been hypothesized that lipofuscin may be the missing link between the factors that are known to be involved in the pathogenesis of AD (oxidative stress, mitochondrial), and the senile plaques that represent its earliest and most specific, microscopically visible structural alterations.

There are other lines of evidence that indicate a major role of lipofuscin in another neuronal degenerative process that is very common in aging: age-related macular degeneration (AMD). Lipofuscin accumulation in the cells of the retina is clearly involved in the pathogenesis of AMD. The accumulation of A2E, the major component of lipofuscin causes apoptosis in the retinal pigment epithelium (RPE), thereby leading to age-related macular degeneration and macular degeneration.

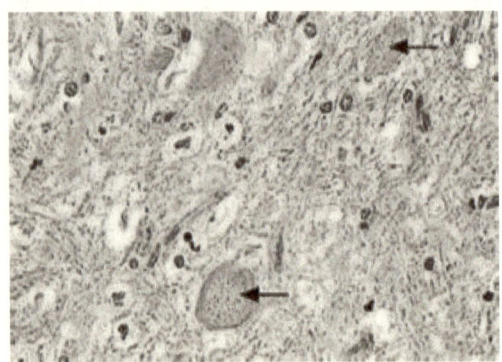

Stargardt's disease is a genetic (hereditary) disorder of the eye that leads to progressive loss of sight. The disease is caused by abnormalities in a gene called

Figure 44: Lipofuscin accumulation in nerve cells (black arrows).

ABCA4, which is responsible for regulating the transport of substances in and out of photoreceptors in the retina. In patients with Stargardt's disease, lipofuscin deposits build up inside the retinal pigment epithelium cells, which become damaged and eventually die.

This leads us to the lipofuscin accumulation hypothesis of aging. The accumulation of oxidized protein with age is due to increased protein damage, decreased oxidized protein degradation and repair, or the combination of both mechanisms leading to increased lipofuscin deposits. As we saw from previous chapters, polyunsaturated fats affect both. Large accumulations of lipofuscin and lipofuscin-like materials eventually lead to cell death. Lipofuscin is often considered in a broader context as one of several forms of undesirable protein aggregations, others sometimes being called ceroids, inclusion bodies, or plaques, depending on their source and composition, common features of neurodegenerative diseases as well as aging

To test this hypothesis, let's examine whether Centrophenoxine (dimethyl aminoethyl p-chlorophenoxyacetate), also known as Meclofenoxate, can affect aging. Centrophenoxine is a dietary supplement developed in 1959 by scientists at the French National Scientific Research Center. Centrophenoxine was originally created as a treatment for Alzheimer's disease, but later was discovered to decrease lipofuscin. Nandy (1968) injected guinea pigs with centrophenoxine for 4-12 weeks. Treated animals showed a notable reduction in lipofuscin inclusions in most parts of the central nervous system, and this reduction was correlated to the duration of treatment. He observed that the granules gradually shrank away leaving an increasingly smaller area of the cell cytoplasm, while concomitantly reducing the activity of lysosomal enzymes. This suggests that the drug is active with respect to lysosomes in the aging process.

Rochschild (1973) treated aged rats with centrophenoxine for eight (8) weeks. There was an observable decrease of pigment of varying intensity between 25-42% depending on the area of the brain studied. Another study by Nandy, looked at the effects of centrophenoxine on the learning and memory of old mice. Old female mice (11-12 months) were treated with centrophenoxine for three months and their learning and memory were tested in a T-maze. The number of attempt to traverse the maze in the 20 treated old mice were the same as those for 20 younger untreated mice. The treated animals learned the task with significantly fewer trials, and also exhibited a reduction of neuronal lipofuscin pigment in both the cerebral cortex and the hippocampus. The results correlate the changes observed in neuronal lipofuscin content with mental performance.

In another intriguing study, centrophenoxine increased the median, mean and maximum survival time from the start of drug administration of male Swiss Webster Albino mice by 29.5% per cent, 27.3% ($P = 0.039$) and 39.7% respectively. This suggests that lowering the lipofuscin content of cells decreases aging.

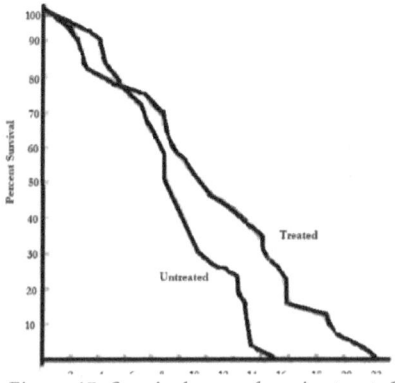

Figure 45: Survival curve for mice treated with 80mg/kg body weight vs untreated controls (months).

Significant differences in lipofuscin density were found between the centrophenoxine treated animals and the control group. Treated mice showed appreciably less pigmentation in myocardial tissue. Brains of control animals appeared darker in color than did those of the drug-treated mice.

Aging

We all age. Yet when it comes to defining aging, or to explain its' mechanism, we are frequently at a loss. Aging is the greatest risk factor for disease, and about two-thirds (2/3) of the population die from age related illnesses. There are four characteristics to aging:

1) it is progressive,
2) endogenous,
3) irreversible
4) deleterious for the individual
5) associated with age-related diseases.

Polyunsaturated Membrane Theory of Aging

There is no lack of theories on aging. Instead of looking at the landscape of theories, we will instead focus on the theory that has garnished the most attention: the "free radical" theory (also known as either the "oxidative stress" or "oxidative damage" theory). The free radial theory is the most accepted explanation of aging and variation in longevity, with much evidence to support it.

Simply defined, the theory states that all living organisms age because cells accumulate free radical damage over time. Aging is associated with:

- an increase in either PUFA content or PI (peroxidation index) of membranes with age,
- an increase in membrane lipid peroxidation with age,
- age-related changes in physicochemical membrane properties.

Evidence shows that as we age, the membrane fatty acid content increases toward peroxidizable PUFAs.

Because the PUFAs are more vulnerable to free radical attack, they experience greater lipid oxidative damage (Figure 46). One of the hallmark of aging is rigidly of cell membranes. Lipid peroxidation products, and peroxidized lipids, are the most likely cause in creating age-related membrane rigidity. The modification of the physical state of the membrane also correlates with the loss of its functioning. Furthermore, as we saw in chapter 5, mitochondrial structure and function are very sensitive to reactive products compounds from lipid peroxidation.

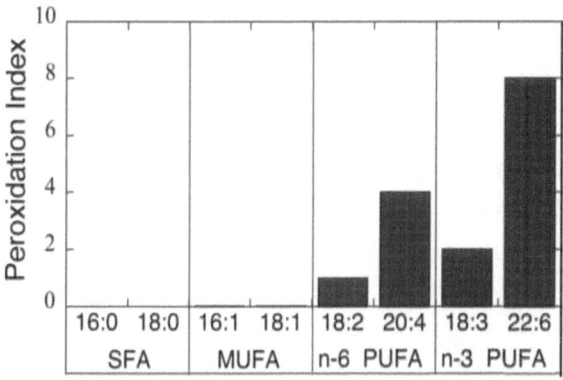

Figure 46: Peroxidation index for saturated fatty acids (SFA), mono-unsaturated fatty acids (MUFA) and polyunsaturated fatty acids (PUFA).

A review of animals with different aging rates have shown that the rate of mitochondrial oxygen radical generation is directly related to the oxidative damage to mitochondrial DNA. In other words, the degree of oxidative damage is inversely correlated with maximum longevity. This is the result of polyunsaturated fats which compose the cellular membrane. And as expected, the degree of unsaturation of tissue fatty acids correlates inversely with maximum longevity. The variation in maximum lifespan among different species is due to the degree of saturation of fats in cellular membranes. Therefore, membrane fatty acid composition is highly correlated with the maximum lifespans of mammals and birds. Long-living mammal species have a more peroxidation resistant membrane composition compared to shorter living similar sized animals. As a species, Homo sapiens owe our exceptional longevity to phospholipids with a particularly peroxidation resistant fatty acid composition.

The range of maximum life span potentials of different species of mammals is great. Therefore, we would expect a different degree of unsaturation of membrane bound fats. Some very small mammals live for less than one (1) year, while some humans have been recorded to live beyond 120 years, making man the longest living species of mammal. It turns out that small mammals also have a higher content of polyunsaturated fats in their membrane than those of larger mammals. For example, the naked mole rat is the longest living rodent known, with a maximum lifespan of greater than 28 years compared to similarly sized mice (3-4 years). While the phospholipid distribution is similar in tissue of both species, DHA-containing phospholipids represent 27-57% of all phospholipids in mice but only 2-6% in naked mole rats. The lower level of DHA-containing phospholipids suggests a lower susceptibility to peroxidative damage in membranes of naked mole rats compared to mice. The membrane composition in mole rats is unchanged with age. Both species have similar amounts of membrane total unsaturated fatty acids; however, mice had 9 times more docosahexaenoic acid (DHA). Because this n-3 PUFA is most susceptible to lipid peroxidation, mole rat membranes are substantially more resistant to oxidative stress than are mice membranes.

There is, of course, considerable longevity variation within species. This difference in life span is seen both between strains of a given species and between individuals within a species. An example of natural variation in longevity is that some wild-derived strains of mice (*Mus musculus*) have been shown to have longer life spans and more delayed maturation than laboratory mice kept under identical environmental conditions. And as expected, long living wild mice strains also have phospholipids with lower peroxidation indices than those of the laboratory mice. Both strains were fed the same diet suggesting a genetic regulation of the differences in membrane composition.

However, the peroxidation-resistant membrane composition can be modified. Caloric restriction is well established as a means of increasing longevity. The use of caloric restriction to manipulate aging was first described in 1935 by McCay *et al*. When rats are subjected to reduced caloric intake, there is a reduction in lipid peroxidation. One might surmise that this is due to a reduction in free radicals from the reduction in metabolic activity. But the action of food restriction could not be attributable to the changes in membrane lipid content nor vitamin E status. Then in 1987, Laganiere and Yu conclusively showed that liver membranes became less susceptible to peroxidation during caloric restriction. These changes in membrane composition are proportional to the degree of caloric restriction, manifesting within one month of beginning of caloric restriction. Restricting calories modified membrane fatty acid composition by increasing linoleic acid and decreasing docosapentaenoic acid phospholipid content.

Pre-natal consumption of omega-3 fatty acids is believed to be beneficial to fetal and infant development by reducing the incidence of preterm births by prolonging pregnancy. Consequently, there is a trend to supplement the expecting mother's diet with large amounts of omega-3 fats. Yet, we also know that either over or under supplementation with omega-3 fats can harm offspring development. As overabundance of omega-3 fats during pregnancy and lactation had adverse effects on life span and sensory/neurological function in adulthood.

Female rats were given one of three diets from the first day of pregnancy through lactation. The three diets were: control omega-3 FA (7% soybean oil), deficient omega-3 FA (7% safflower oil), and excess omega-3 FA (7% fish oil). The rat pups in the excess group had slowed neural transmission times and had postnatal growth restriction. In addition, the offspring had shorter life spans compared to their control and omega-3 deficient rats. Therefore, excess amounts of omega-3 FA during pregnancy and lactation adversely affects the offspring's neural transmission times and postnatal thriving.

Epidemiology

There has been a dramatic increase in life expectancy during the 20th century. Most babies born in 1900 did not live past age 50. In contrast, life expectancy is close to 90 years in Monaco. In fact, life expectancy in the top 10 countries exceeds 82 years (Figure 47). The change in longevity is part of a major transition in public

Rank	Country	Years
1	Monaco	89.52
2	Japan	84.74
3	Singapore	84.68
4	Macau	84.51
5	San Marino	83.24
6	Iceland	82.97
7	Hong Kong	82.86
8	Andorra	82.72
9	Switzerland	82.50
10	Guernsey	82.47
11	Israel	82.27
18	Canada	81.76
43	United States	79.68

Figure 47: Average life expectancy for 2015. The country with the highest life expectancy is Monaco at 89.52 years; the country with the lowest life expectancy is Chad at just 49.81 years.

health spending across the globe. In modern societies, most people live past middle age with death concentrated in the elderly. However, in this has not always been the case with deaths occurring at every age in the past.

The changes in longevity is due to many factors including a decline in fertility, a decline in infant mortality, a shift in diseases from communicable diseases to chronic diseases, and an overall improvement in disease treatment. But with the aforementioned variables, it is near impossible to tease out the overall effect of diet on aging. As we saw in the preceding chapters, there is a large variability in cancer, obesity and heart disease, and this variability impacts the overall longevity numbers.

There are isolated areas in a number of societies where there are large number of individuals over 90 years of age. Some of the oldest people on the face of the earth live in the Caucasus. The most famous was Shirali Muslimov of Azerbaijan, who died on September 2, 1973, at the undocumented age of 168. Azerbaijan has one of the highest rates of longevity in the world. Azerbaijan recorded 5.8% of the population over the age of 65 in the 2012 census. The Azerbaijan diet includes daily consumption of yogurt and garlic while meat is available only in the winter. Azerbaijanis are fond of saturated fat consisting of lamb, mutton and sheep fat, with the main source of animal fat from dairy products. The typical diet of Azerbaijani villagers consists primarily of eggs, cheese, butter, yogurt, milk, curds (shor), sour cream, bread, various vegetables, fruits and herbs. Polyunsaturated fat is virtually non-existent in the diet.

Okinawa is made up of a few dozen, small islands in the southern half of the Nansei Shoto island chain, about 640 kilometers south of Japan's Kyushu island. Elderly Okinawans have among the lowest mortality rates in the world, delaying, or sometimes escaping, the chronic diseases of aging including dementia, cardiovascular disease (coronary heart disease and stroke) and cancer. They enjoy not only what may be the world's longest life expectancy but the world's longest health expectancy. Their diet, compared to other Japanese islands indicate Okinawans consumed less polyunsaturated fat (4.8% of calories vs. 8%), and less overall caloric intake.

Throughout this book, we have studied the impact of polyunsaturated fats on multiple chronic disease and the protective role of the elimination of dietary polyunsaturated fatty acids. Therefore, a diet of reduced polyunsaturated/saturated fat ratio would be expected to increased human longevity. A population-based, prospective study, was conducted in one of the eight centers of the Italian Longitudinal Study on Aging (ILSA). They investigated the possible role of monounsaturated, polyunsaturated, and other selected food groups in protecting against all-causes mortality following an 8.5-year follow-up. A total of 278 persons agreed to participate in the survey. There were 91 deaths recorded. A diet enriched with monounsaturated fatty acids was associated with an increase of survival. A higher unsaturated fatty acid to saturated ratio correlated with an increased total mortality, while no effect about other selected food groups were found.

Mitochondrial Decay in Aging

Our mitochondria are essential to life. They are involved in energy production, programmed cell death and regulation of the production of reactive oxygen species. As we saw in chapter 5, there are several ways in which unsaturated fats can disrupt mitochondrial function. Overall lipid content of the cardiolipin molecule can be altered with the dietary consumption of PUFAs. The lipid structure of cardiolipin is dependent on dietary fats, and any disturbance of the cardiolipin profile will result in mitochondrial dysfunction. In addition, high amounts of polyunsaturated oil will overwhelm the antioxidant system leading to more peroxidation of mitochondrial structures.

There is a large number of comparative studies that support the notion that mitochondrial membrane composition is linked to lifespan. These studies have revealed that lipid unsaturation ratios actually correlate with lifespan. Mitochondrial function declines with age. This decline is expressed as a decrease in membrane fluidity as well as a decrease in function of cardiolipin. The reactive oxygen species (ROS) created by the mitochondria appear to be the major source of the oxidative products that accumulate with age. These ROS in turn cause the oxidative damage seen in aging. The damaged mitochondria produce significantly less energy, due in part to the accumulation of polyunsaturated fatty acids. Because of their wide range of functions, mitochondria have been strongly implicated in aging and longevity. Many studies lead to the conclusion that aging, and decreased lifespan, are associated with high reactive oxygen species production by mitochondria, increased mitochondrial DNA and protein damage, as well as with changes in the fatty acid composition of mitochondrial membranes.

The mitochondria have a potent self-repair system, with a capacity to fuse with sister mitochondria, and divide. During fusion, mitochondria exchange material with other mitochondria. With division, the mitochondria split into two daughter mitochondria. With both fusion and division, mitochondria can renew themselves by dilution of mitochondria damage. If this renewal mechanism worked perfectly, the cell would remain vital and possibly halt aging. However, over time, peroxidation of unsaturated mitochondrial membranes leads to a slow accumulation of poorly functioning mitochondria.

In chapter 5, we looked at the activities of electron transport chain and its relationship to mitochondria function. The eelectron transport chain resides on the inner membrane of the mitochondria and is the basis for extracting energy. The electron transport chain consists of a separated series of chemical reactions where electrons are transferred to a series of complexes called respiratory complex I to IV. This cascading series of reactions ultimately involves oxygen binding to oxygen to form water. The electron transport chain is essential to life which is why blocking it with cyanide is immediately fatal. In aging, activities of respiratory complexes I and IV are significantly decrease with the age compared to the activity of the same enzymes in young animals. The fatty acid composition of muscle homogenates of old rats differed from that of young animals as by a reduced content of saturated and monosaturated fats (myristic & oleic acids) and an increase in polyunsaturated fats (dihomo-γ-linolenic, arachidonic, and docosahexaenoic acids). Oral supplementation of the old rats with hydrogenated peanut oil (saturated fat) completely restored the activity of complex IV and increased the activity of complex I to 80% of the value observed in muscles of young animals. Adding saturated fat to the diet of old rats reduced the polyunsaturated fats (dihomo-γ-linolenic, arachidonic, eicosapentaenoic, docosapentaenoic, and docosahexaenoic acids) in mitochondrial membranes relative to young rats. This suggest that the mitochondrial dysfunction that occurs with aging can be reduced by replacing polyunsaturated fats in the diet with saturated fat.

Myocardial (heart muscle) aging, can lead to circulatory dysfunction, and is an important contributor to overall mortality at old age. In the cardiac muscle (myocyte), mitochondria and lysosomes suffer remarkable age-related alterations. These mitochondrial changes include structural changes and enlargement, while lysosomes, accumulate lipofuscin as previously discussed.

Since the heart is constantly contracting, you would expect that the myocardial cells contain an abundance of mitochondria to meet the energy demand. And with the increase in mitochondrial population is an overall increase in cardiolipin compared to other skeletal muscle. As discussed in chapter 5, cardiolipin is a phospholipid containing predominately linoleic acid. And with aging we see a change in the cardiolipin molecule over time with the consumption of polyunsaturated fats in the diet.

Lee, *et.al.* (2006) measured the fatty acid concentration of cardiolipin in the hearts of rats aged 4, 12 and

24 months. They observed the concentration of linoleic acid was decreased in 24-month-old rats versus 4-month-old rats. The concentrations of arachidonic and docosahexaenoic acid were increased in 24-month-old rats. These results demonstrate that cardiolipin remodeling occurs with aging, specifically an increase in highly unsaturated fatty acids. In addition, the heart mitochondrial content of cardiolipin, is markedly reduced (approximately 40%) in aged rats. This reduced mitochondrial cytochrome c oxidase activity in aged animals is due to a specific decrease in the cardiolipin content.

And so, it seems we have gone full circle. Perhaps the greatest problem with polyunsaturated fats are their effect on the mitochondria. Without the metabolic engine of the cell, the other consequences of vegetable oils in the diet seem negligible. The process of polyunsaturated fats being substituted in the membranes of this organelle is the molecular equivalent of sand in the gears. Mitochondria become dysfunctional and enlarge, leading to a cascade of problems including cancer, heart disease, and aging. I prefer my mitochondria healthy!

About the Author

Thomas Copmann, MS., PhD, has authored over 50 peer-reviewed articles. He holds an MS in Endocrinology and a PhD in Physiology and Post-Doctoral training in Neuroendocrinology. He is currently a consultant to the pharmaceutical industry. He has been active on editorial boards, advisory boards and as a member of boards of directors. He is the former Chair of the Commission on Drugs for Rare Diseases; former Advisor to the National Vaccine Advisory Board. He has served as a scientific advisor to the White House.

End Notes

Chapter 1: The Elegant Complexity of Fats

Gurr, MI. and Harwood, JL. Fatty acid structure and metabolism. In: Gurr MI and Harwood JL (eds) Lipid Biochemistry, An Introduction. London: Chapman and Hall, 1991.

Rustan, AC. And Drevon, CA. Fatty Acids: Structures and Properties. Encyclopedia of Life Sciences, John Wiley & Sons, Ltd, 2005

Chapter 2: Seed Oils

Jung, M.Y. Yoon, S.H., Min, D.B. Effects of Processing Steps on the Contents of Minor Components and Oxidation of Soybean Oil. *Journal of American Oil Chemists ' Society.* 66: 118- 120, 1989.

Rossell, J.B., Kochhar, S.P. and Jawad, I.M. Chemical Changes in Soy Oil During High Temperature Processing. Proceedings Second ASA Symp. Soyabean Processing, Antwerp, 1981.

Segers, J.C. and van de Sande, R. Degumming Theory and Practice. Proceedings AOCS World Conference on Edible Fats and Oils Processing. Maastricht pp 88-83, 1988.

Vossen P. Olive Oil: History, Production, and Characteristics of the World's Classic Oils *HortScience* 42(5):1093-1100, 2007.

Chapter 3: Lipid Peroxidation

Ayala, A., Muñoz, MF., and Argüelles, S. Lipid Peroxidation: Production, Metabolism, and Signaling Mechanisms of Malondialdehyde and 4-Hydroxy-2-Nonenal. *Oxid Med Cell Longev*. 2014;2014.

Burcham, PC. Genotoxic Lipid Peroxidation Products: Their DNA Damaging Properties and Role in Formation of Endogenous DNA Adducts. *Mutagenesis*. (13)3: 287-305, 1998.

Dalleau, S., Baradat, M., Gue'raud, F., and Huc, L. Cell Death and Diseases Related to Oxidative Stress: 4-hydroxynonenal (HNE) in the Balance. *Cell Death and Differentiation*. 20, 1615-1630, 2013.

Dalle-Donne, I., Rossi, R., Colombo, R., Giustarini, D.,

and Milzani, A. Biomarkers of Oxidative Damage in Human Disease. *Clinical Chemistry*. 52:4 601-623, 2006.

Doureradjou, P. and Koner, BC. Effect of Different Cooking Vessels on Heat Induced Lipid Peroxidation of Different Edible Oils. *Journal of Food Biochemistry*. (32) 6: 740-751, 2008.

Esterbauer, H., Jurgens, G., Quehenberger, O., and Koller, QE. Autoxidation of Human Low Density Lipoprotein: Loss of Polyunsaturated Fatty Acids and Vitamin E and Generation of Aldehydes. *J Lipid Res*. 28: 495-509, 1987.

Fang, J., Vaca, CE., 4, Valsta, LM., and Mutanen, M. Determination of DNA Adducts of Malonaldehyde in Humans: Effects of Dietary Fatty Acid Composition. *Carcinogenesis*. (17)5: 1035-1040, 1996.

Gago-Dominguez, M., Jiang, X., and Castelao, JE. Lipid Peroxidation, Oxidative Stress Genes and Dietary Factors in Breast Cancer Protection: a Hypothesis. *Breast Cancer Research*. 9:201, 2007.

Galano, JM., Mas, E., Barden, A., Mori, TA., Signorini, C., De Felice, C., Barrett, A., Opere, C., Pinot, E., Schwedhelm, E., Benndorf, R., Roy, J., Le Guennec, JY., Oger, C., and Durand, T. Isoprostanes and Neuroprostanes: Total Synthesis, Biological Activity and Biomarkers of Oxidative Stress in Humans. *Prostaglandins*. 04(003), 2013.

Girotti, AW. Lipid Hydroperoxide Generation, Turnover, and Effector Action in Biological Systems. *J Lipid Res*. 39: 1529-1542, 1998.

Gueraud, F., Atalay, M., Bresgen, N., Cipak, A., Eckl, PM., Huc, L., Jouanin, I., Siems, W., and Uchida, K. Chemistry and Biochemistry of Lipid Peroxidation Products. *Free Radical Research.* 44(10): 1098-1124, 2010.

Halvorsen, BL., and Blomhoff, R. Determination of Lipid Oxidation Products in Vegetable Oils and Marine Omega-3 Supplements *Food & Nutrition Research.* (55) 5792, 2011.

Jones, R. and Mann, T. Toxicity of Exogenous Fatty Acid Peroxides Towards Spermatozoa. *J Reprod Fert.* 50, 255-260, 1977.

Leong XF., Ng CY., Jaarin K., and Mustafa, MR. Effects of Repeated Heating of Cooking Oils on Antioxidant Content and Endothelial Function. *Austin J Pharmacol Ther.* (3)2: 1-7, 2015.

Lai, C., , Jaakkola, JJ., Chuang, C., Liou, S., Lung, S., Loh C., Yu, D., and Strickland, PT. Exposure to Cooking Oil Fumes and Oxidative Damages: A Longitudinal Study in Chinese Military Cooks. *Expo Sci Environ Epidemiol.* 23(1): 94-100, 2013.

Moore, S.A., Humphreys, E., Friesen, M.D., Shuker, D.E.G., and Bingham, S.A. The Effect of n-6 Polyunsaturated Fatty Acid on Blood Levels of Malondialdehyde-Deoxyguanosine Adducts in Human Subjects. *The Open Biomarkers J.* 1: 28-35, 2008.

Nair, J., Vaca, CE., Velic, I., Mutanen, M., Valsta, LM., and Bartsch, H. High Dietary w-6 Polyunsaturated Fatty Acids Drastically Increase The Formulation of Etheno-

DNA Base Adducts in White Blood Cells of Female Subjects. *Cancer Epidemiology, Biomarkers & Prevention.* 6: 597-601, 1997.

Negre-Salvayre, A., Coatrieux, C., Ingueneau, C., and Salvayre, R. Advanced Lipid Peroxidation End Products in Oxidative Damage to Proteins. Potential Role in Diseases and Therapeutic Prospects for the Inhibitors *Brit J of Pharm.* 153, 6-20, 2008.

Romero, FJ., Bosch-Morell, F., Romero, MJ., Jareflo, EJ., Romero, B., Marin, N., and Roma, J. Lipid Peroxidation Products and Antioxidants in Human Disease. *Environ Health Perspect.* 106(Suppl 5):1229-1234, 1998.

Sadoudi R., Ammouche A. and Ali Ahmed, D. Effect of Ingestion of Thermally Oxidized Sunflower Oil on the Fatty Acid Composition and Histological Alteration of Rat Liver and Adipose Tissue in Development *Afr J Agric Res.* 8(24): 3107-3112, 2013.

Schlame, M., Horvatht, L., and Vigh, L. Relationship Between Lipid Saturation and Lipid-protein Interaction in Liver Mitochondria Modified by Catalytic Hydrogenation with Reference to Cardiolipin Molecular Species. *Biochem J.* 265, 79-85, 1990.

Shamberger, RJ., Shamberger, BA., and Willis, CE. Malonaldehyde Content of Food. *J Nutr.* 107: 1404-1409, 1977.

Song, JH., Fujimoto, K., and Miyazawa, T. Polyunsaturated (n-3) Fatty Acids Susceptible to Peroxidation Are Increased in Plasma and Tissue Lipids of Rats Fed Docosahexaenoic Acid-Containing Oils. *J Nutr.* 130: 3028-

3033, 2000.

Tak Yee Aw, Biliary Glutathione Promotes the Mucosal Metabolism of Luminal Peroxidized Lipids by Rat Small Intestine In Vivo. *J Clin Invest*. 94: 1218-1225, 1994.

Trevisan, M., Browne, R., Ram, M., Muti, P., Freudenheim, J., Carosella, AM., and Armstrong, D. Correlates of Markers of Oxidative Status in the General Population. *Am J Epidemiol*. 154:348-56, 2001.

Uchida, K., Kanematsu, M., Morimitsu, Y., Osawa, T., Noguchi, N., and Niki, E. Acrolein Is a Product of Lipid Peroxidation Reaction *J Biol Chem*. 273(26): 16058-16066, 1998.

Uddin, I., Ahmad, S., Ul Haq, I., Nawab, S., and Uddin, M. Thermally Oxidized Corn Oil Adversely Affects Serum Biochemistry, Blood Hematology and Liver Histopathology of Rabbits. *Euro Academic Res*. 3(2), 2015.

Varady, J., Gessner, DK., Most, E., Eder, K., and Ringseis, R. Dietary Moderately Oxidized Oil Activates the Nrf2 Signaling Pathway in the Liver of Pigs. *Lipids in Health and Disease*. (11)31, 2012.

Chapter 4: Arteriosclerosis and Cardiovascular Disease

Abramson, J. and Wright, JM. Are Lipid-lowering Guidelines Evidence-based? *Lancet*. 369(9557): 168-9, 2007.

Anderson, KM., Castelli, WP., and Levy, D. Cholesterol and Mortality: 30 Years of Follow-up From the Framingham Study. *JAMA*. 257(16):2176-2180, 1987.

Armingohar, Z., Jørgensen, J.J., Kristoffersen, AK., Abesha-Belay, E., and Olsen, I. Bacteria and Bacterial DNA in Atherosclerotic Plaque and Aneurysmal Wall Biopsies From Patients with and Without Periodontitis. *J Oral Microbiol*. 6: 23408, 2014.

Bonanome, A., Pagnan, A., Biffanti, S., Opportuno, A., Sorgato, F., Dorella, M., Maiorino, M. and Ursini, F. Effect of Dietary Monounsaturated and Polyunsaturated Fatty Acids on the Susceptibility of Plasma Low Density Lipoproteins to Oxidative Modification. *Arteriosclerosis and Thrombosis*. 12:529-533, 1992.

Boulanger, CM., Amabile, N., and Tedgui, T. Circulating Microparticles: A Potential Prognostic Marker for Atherosclerotic Vascular Disease. *Hypertension*. 48:180-186, 2006.

Barski, OA., Xie, Z., Baba, SP., Sithu, SS., Agarwal, A., Cai, J., Bhatnagar, A., and Srivastava, S. Dietary Carnosine Prevents Early Atherosclerotic Lesion Formation in ApoE-null Mice. *Arterioscler Thromb Vasc Biol*. 33(6), 2013.

Barter, PJ., Caulfield, M., Eriksson, M., Grundy, SM., Kastelein, JJ., Komajda, M., Lopez-Sendon, J., Mosca, L., Tardif, JC., Waters, DD., Shear, CL., Revkin, JH., Buhr, KA., Fisher, MR., Tall, AR., Brewer, B.; ILLUMINATE Investigators. Effects of Torcetrapib in Patients at High Risk for Coronary Events. *N Engl J Med*. 357(21): 2109-

22, 2007.

Chapple, SJ., Cheng, X., and Mann, GE. Effects of 4-hydroxynonenal on Vascular Endothelial and Smooth Muscle Cell Redox Signaling and Function in Health and Disease. *Redox Biology*. 1:319-331, 2013.

Chowdhury, R., Warnakula, S., Kunutsor, S., Crowe, F., Ward, HA., Johnson, L., Franco, OH., Butterworth, AS., Forouhi, NG., Thompson, SG., Khaw, KT., Mozaffarian, D., Danesh, J., and Di Angelantonio, E. Association of Dietary, Circulating, and Supplement Fatty Acids with Coronary Risk: A Systematic Review and Meta-analysis. *Ann Intern Med*. 160(9):658, 2014.

Contois, JH., McConnell, JP., Sethi, AA., Csako, G., Devaraj, S., Hoefner, DM., and Warnick, GR. Apolipoprotein B and Cardiovascular Disease Risk: Position Statement from the AACC Lipoproteins and Vascular Diseases Division Working Group on Best Practices. *Clin Chem*. 55:3 407-419, 2009.

Dessi, M., Noce, A., Bertucci, P., Manca di Villahermosa, S., Zenobi, R., Castagnola, V., Addessi, E., and Di Daniele, N. Atherosclerosis, Dyslipidemia, and Inflammation: The Significant Role of Polyunsaturated Fatty Acids. *ISRN Inflamm*. 2013:191823, 2013.

Esterbauer, H., Jurgens, G., Quehenberger, O., and Koller, E. Autoxidation of Human Low Density Lipoprotein: Loss of Polyunsaturated Fatty Acids and Vitamin E and Generation of Aldehydes. *J Lipid Res*. 28: 495-509, 1987.

Felton, CV., Crook, D., Davies, MJ., and Oliver, MF. Dietary Polyunsaturated Fatty Acids and Composition of Human Aortic Plaques. *Lancet*. 344(8931):1195-6, 1994.

Galvao, TF., Brown, BH., Hecker, PA., O'Connell, KA., O'Shea,. KM, Sabbah, HN., Rastogi, S., Daneault, C., Des Rosiers, C., and Stanley, WC. High Intake of Saturated Fat, but not Polyunsaturated Fat, Improves Survival in Heart Failure Despite Persistent Mitochondrial Defects. *Cardiovasc Res*. 93(1): 24-32, 2012.

Gniwotta, C., Morrow, JD., Roberts, LJ., and Kühn, H. Prostaglandin F2-like Compounds, F2-isoprostanes, are Present in Increased Amounts in Human Atherosclerotic Lesions. *Arterioscler Thromb Vasc Biol*. 17(11):3236-41, 1997.

Glushakova, O., Kosugi, T., Roncal, C., Mu, W., Marcelo Heinig, M., Cirillo, P., Sánchez-Lozada, LG., Johnson, RJ., and Nakagawa, T. Fructose Induces the Inflammatory Molecule ICAM-1 in Endothelial Cells. *J Am Soc Nephrol*. 19(9): 1712-1720, 2008.

Grenon, SM., Aguado-Zuniga, J., Hatton, JP., Owens, CD., Conte, MS., and Hughes-Fulford, M. Effects of Fatty Acids on Endothelial Cells: Inflammation and Monocyte Adhesion. *J Sur. Res*. 177(1), 2012.

Harcombe, Z., Baker, JS., Cooper, SM., Davies, B., Sculthorpe, N., DiNicolantonio, JJ., and Grace, F. Evidence from Randomized Controlled Trials Did Not Support the Introduction of Dietary Fat Guidelines in 1977 and 1983: A Systematic Review and Meta-analysis. *Open Heart*. 2:e000196, 2015.

Krauss, RM. Atherogenic Lipoprotein Phenotype and Diet-Gene Interactions. *J Nutr*. 131:340S-343S, 2001.

Lawrence, GD. Dietary Fats and Health: Dietary Recommendations in the Context of Scientific Evidence. *Adv Nutr*. 4: 294-302, 2013.

Leren, P. The Effect of Plasma-cholesterol-lowering Diet in Male Survivors of Myocardial Infarction. A Controlled Clinical Trial. *Bull N Y Acad Med*. 44(8): 1012-20, 1968.

Martin, SS., Qasim, AN., Mehta, NN., Wolfe, M., Terembula, K., Schwartz, S., Iqbal, N., Schutta, M., Bagheri, R., and Reilly, MP. Apolipoprotein B but not LDL Cholesterol Is Associated With Coronary Artery Calcification in Type 2 Diabetic Whites. *Diabetes*. 58:1887-1892, 2009.

Martinet, W., and De Meyer, GRY. Autophagy in Atherosclerosis. A Cell Survival and Death Phenomenon With Therapeutic Potential. *Circ Res*. 104:304-317, 2009.

Mozaffarian, D., Rimm, EB., and Herrington, DM. Dietary Fats, Carbohydrate, and Progression of Coronary Atherosclerosis in Postmenopausal Women. *Am J Clin Nutr*. 80:1175-84, 2004.

Nakazato, R., Gransar, H., Berman, DS., Cheng, VY., Lin, FY., Achenbach, S., Al-Mallah, M., Budoff, MJ., Cademartiri, F., Callister, TQ., Chang, HJ., Cury, RC., Chinnaiyan, K., Chow, BJ., Delago, A., Hadamitzky, M., Hausleiter, J., Kaufmann, P., Maffei, E., Raff, G., Shaw, LJ., Villines, TC., Dunning, A., Feuchtner, G., Kim, YJ.,

Leipsic, J., and Min, JK. Statins use and Coronary Artery Plaque Composition: Results from the International Multicenter CONFIRM Registry. *Atherosclerosis*. 225(1): 148-53, 2012.

Nissen, SE., Tardif, JC., Nicholls, SJ., Revkin, JH., Shear, CL., Duggan, WT., Ruzyllo, W., Bachinsky, WB., Lasala, GP., Tuzcu, EM.; ILLUSTRATE Investigators. Effect of Torcetrapib on the Progression of Coronary Atherosclerosis. *N Engl J Med*. 356:1304-1316, 2007.

Nozue, T., Yamamoto, S., Tohyama, S., Fukui, K., Umezawa, S., Onishi, Y., Kunishima, T, Sato, A., Nozato, T.,Miyake, S., Takeyama, Y., Morino, Y., Yamauchi, T., Muramatsu, T., Kiyoshi Hibi, K., Terashima, M., and Michishita, I. Effects of Serum n-3 to n-6 Polyunsaturated Fatty Acids Ratios on Coronary Atherosclerosis in Statin-Treated Patients With Coronary Artery Disease. *Am J Cardiol*. 1:6-11, 2013.

Ouchi, N., Kobayashi, H., Kihara, S., Kumada, M., Sato, K., Inoue, T., Funahashi, T., and Walsh, K. Adiponectin Stimulates Angiogenesis by Promoting Cross-talk Between AMP-activated Protein Kinase and Akt Signaling in Endothelial Cells. *J Biol Chem*. 279(2): 1304-1309, 2004.

Penumetcha, M., Khan, N., and Parthasarathy, S. Dietary Oxidized Fatty Acids: An Atherogenic Risk? *J Lipid Res*. 41:1473-1480, 2000.

Petursson, H., Sigurdsson, JA., Bengtsson, C., Nilsen, TI., and Getz, L. Is the Use of Cholesterol in Mortality Risk Algorithms in Clinical Guidelines Valid? Ten Years Prospective Data from the Norwegian HUNT 2 Study. *J*

Eval Clin Pract. 18(1):159-68, 2012.

Prior, IA., Davidson, F., Salmond, CE., Czochanska, Z. Cholesterol, Coconuts and Diet on Polynesian Atolls: A Natural Experiment: The Pukapuka and Tokelau Island Studies. *Am J Clin Nutr*. 34:1552-1561, 1981.

Reaven, P., Parthasarathy, S., Grasse, BJ., Miller, E., Almazan, F., Mattson, FH., Khoo, JC., Steinberg., D, and Witztum, JL. Feasibility of Using an Oleate-rich Diet to Reduce the Susceptibility of Low-density Lipoprotein to Oxidative Modification in Humans. *Am J Clin Nutr*. 54(4):701-6, 1991.

Ramsden, CE., Hibbeln, JR., and Majchrzak-Hong, SF. All PUFAs are not Created Equal: Absence of CHD Benefit Specific to Linoleic Acid in Randomized Controlled Trials and Prospective Observational Cohorts. World Rev. *Nutr Diet*. 102: 30-43, 2011.

Reaven,P., Parthasarathy,S., Grasse,BJ., Miller,E., Steinberg,D., and Witztum, JL. Effects of Oleate-rich and Linoleate-rich Diets on the Susceptibility of Low Density Lipoprotein to Oxidative Modification

in Mildly Hypercholesterolemic Subjects. *J Clin Invest*. 91:668-676, 1993.

Rouaki, F., Mazari, A., Kanane, A., Errahmani, MB., and Ammouche, A. Cardiotoxicity Induced by Dietary Oxidized Sunflower Oil in Rats: Pro- and Antioxidant Effects of α-tocopherol. *Int J Vitam Nutr Res*. 83(6):367-76, 2013.

Rose, GA., Thomson, WB., and Williams, RT. Corn Oil in Treatment of Ischaemic Heart Disease. *Brit med J*. 1: 1531-1533, 1995.

Rosenfeld, ME., Palinski, W., Yla-Herttuala,S., Butler,S., and Witztum, JL. Distribution of Oxidation Specific Lipid-Protein Adducts and Apolipoprotein B in Atherosclerotic Lesions of Varying Severity from WHHL Rabbits. *Arteriosclerosis*. 10:336-349, 1990.

Saremi, A., Bahn, G., and Reaven, PD, Progression of Vascular Calcification Is Increased With Statin Use in the Veterans Affairs Diabetes Trial (VADT). *Diabetes Care*. 35: 2390–2392, 2012

Scandinavian Simvastatin Survival Study Group. Randomised trial of cholesterol lowering in 4444 patients with coronary heart disease: the Scandinavian Simvastatin Survival Study (4S). *Lancet*. 344(8934): 1383-9, 1994.

Silaste, ML., Rantala, M., Alfthan, G., Aro, A., Witztum, JL., Kesaniemi, YA., and Horkko, S. Changes in Dietary Fat Intake Alter Plasma Levels of Oxidized Low-Density Lipoprotein and Lipoprotein(a). *Arterioscler Thromb Vasc Biol*. 24:498-503, 2004.

Schwartz, GG., Olsson, AG., Abt, M.,Ballantyne, CM., Barter, PJ., Brumm, J., Chaitman, BR., Holme, IM., Kallend, D., Leiter, LA., Leitersdorf, E., McMurray, JJV., Mundl, H., Nicholls, SJ., Shah, PK., Tardif, JC., and Wright, RS. Effects of Dalcetrapib in Patients with a Recent Acute Coronary Syndrome. *N Engl J Med*. 367:2089-99, 2012.

Takahashi, R., Goto, T., Oe, T., and Lee, SH. Angiotensin II Modification by Decomposition Products of Linoleic Acid-derived Lipid Hydroperoxide. *Chem Biol. Interact.* 239: 87-99, 2015.

Waddington, EI., Croft, KD., Sienuarine, K., Latham, B., and Puddey IB. Fatty acid Oxidation Products in Human Atherosclerotic Plaque: An Analysis of Clinical and Histopathological Correlates. *Atherosclerosis.* 167(1): 111-20, 2003.

Williams, PT., Krauss, RM., Vranizan, KM., Stefanick, ML., Wood, PDS., and Lindgren, FT. Associations of Lipoproteins and Apolipoproteins With Gradient Gel Electrophoresis Estimates of High Density Lipoprotein Subfractions in Men and Women. *Arteriosclerosis and Thrombosis.* 12:332-430, 1992.

Yam, D., Eliraz, A., and Berry, EM. Diet and Disease-The Israeli Paradox: Possible Dangers of a High Omega-6 Polyunsaturated Fatty Acid Diet. *Isr J Med Sci.* 32(11):1134-43, 1996.

Zhong, H., Lu, J., Xia, L., Zhu, M., and Yin, H. Formation of Electrophilic Oxidation Products from Mitochondrial Cardiolipin in-vitro and in vivo in the Context of Apoptosis and Atherosclerosis. *Redox Biol.* 2:878-883, 2014.

Chapter 5: Polyunsaturated Fats and Cancer

Alsheikh-Ali, AA., Maddukuri, PV., Han, H., and Karas, RH. Effect of the Magnitude of Lipid Lowering on

Risk of Elevated Liver Enzymes, Rhabdomyolysis, and Cancer: Insights from Large Randomized Statin Trials. *J Am Coll Cardiol*. 31;50(5):409-18, 2007.

Artwohl, M., Roden, M., Waldhäusl, W., Freudenthaler, A., Baumgartner-Parzer, SM. Free Fatty Acids Trigger Apoptosis and Inhibit Cell Cycle Progression in Human Vascular Endothelial Cells. *FASEB J*. 18(1):146-8, 2004.

Azrad, M., Turgeon, C., and Demark-Wahnefried, W. Current Evidence Linking Polyunsaturated Fatty Acids with Cancer Risk and Progression. *Frontiers in Oncology - Cancer Molecular Targets and Therapeutics*, 3(224) 4-12, 2013.

Bartsch, H.,, Nair, J., and Owen, RW. Dietary Polyunsaturated Fatty Acids and Cancers of the Breast and Colorectum: Emerging Evidence for their Role as Risk Modifiers. *Carcinogenesis*. 20(12): 2209-18, 1999.

Basova, LV., Kurnikov, IV., Wang, L., Ritov, VB., Belikova,. NA, Vlasova, II., Pacheco, AA., Winnica, DE., Peterson, J., Bayir, H., Waldeck, DH., and Kagan, VE. Cardiolipin Switch in Mitochondria: Shutting Off the Reduction of Cytochrome C and Turning on the Peroxidase Activity. *Biochem*. 46(11): 3423-34, 2007.

Berquin, IM., Min, Y., Wu, R., Wu, J., Perry, D., Cline, JM., Thomas, MJ., Thornburg, T., Kulik, G., Smith, A., Edwards, IJ., D'Agostino, R., Zhang, H., Wu, H., Kang, JX., and Chen, YQ. Modulation of Prostate Cancer Genetic Risk by Omega-3 and Umega-6 Fatty Acids. *J Clin Invest*. 117(7): 1866-75, 2007.

Brasky, TM., Till, C., White, E., Neuhouser, ML., Song,

X., Goodman, P., Thompson, IM., King, IB., Albanes, D., and Kristal, AR. Serum Phospholipid Fatty Acids and Prostate Cancer Risk: Results from the Prostate Cancer Prevention Trial. *Am J Epidemiol*. 173(12):1429-39, 2011.

Broitman, SA., Vitale, JJ., Vavrousek-Jakuba, E., and Gottlieb, LS. Polyunsaturated Fat, Cholesterol and Large Bowel Tumorigenesis. *Cancer*. 40(5 Suppl):2455-63, 1977.

Chen, JJ. and Yu, BP. Alterations in Mitochondrial Membrane Fluidity by Lipid Peroxidation Products. *Free Radic Biol Med*. 17(5): 411-8, 1994.

Chicco, AJ. and Sparagna, GC. Role of Cardiolipin Alterations in Mitochondrial Dysfunction and Disease. *Am J Physiol Cell Physiol*. 292: C33-C44, 2007.

Chole, RH., Patil, RN., Basak, A., Palandurkar, K., and Bhowate, R. Estimation of Serum Malondialdehyde in Oral Cancer and Precancer and its Association with Healthy Individuals, Gender, Alcohol, and Tobacco Abuse. *J Cancer Res Ther*. 6(4):487-91, 2010.

Colin H. Cortie, CH. and Else, PL. Dietary Docosahexaenoic Acid (22:6) Incorporates into Cardiolipin at the Expense of Linoleic Acid (18:2): Analysis and Potential Implications. *Biochem*. 46(11): 3423-34, 2007.

Cortie, CH. and Else, PL. Dietary Docosahexaenoic Acid (22:6) Incorporates into Cardiolipin at the Expense of Linoleic Acid (18:2):

Analysis and Potential Implications. *Int J Mol Sci*. 13:

15447-15463, 2012.

Crowe, FL., Allen, NE., Appleby, PN., Overvad, K., Aardestrup, IV., Johnsen, NF., Tjønneland, A., Linseisen, J., Kaaks, R., Boeing, H., Kröger, J., Trichopoulou, A., Zavitsanou, A., Trichopoulos, D., Sacerdote, C., Palli, D., Tumino, R., Agnoli, C., Kiemene,y LA., Bueno-de-Mesquita, HB., Chirlaque, MD., Ardanaz, E., Larrañaga, N., Quirós, JR., Sánchez, MJ., González, CA., Stattin, P., Hallmans, G., Bingham, S., Khaw ,KT., Rinaldi, S., Slimani, N., Jenab, M., Riboli, E., and Key, TJ. Fatty Acid Composition of Plasma Phospholipids and Risk of Prostate Cancer in a Case-control Analysis Nested within the European Prospective Investigation into Cancer and Nutrition. *Am J Clin Nutr*. 88(5): 1353-63, 2008.

Davila, AF., and Zamorano P. Mitochondria and the Evolutionary Roots of Cancer. *Phys Biol*. 10(2):026008, 2013.

Ding, EL. and Hu, FB. Cancer and Cholesterol: Understanding the V-shaped Association in Patients with Diabetes. *CMAJ*. 179(5): 403-404, 2008.

Fauser, JK., Matthews, GM., Cummins, AG., and Howarth, GS. Induction of Apoptosis by the Medium-chain Length Fatty Acid Lauric Acid in Colon Cancer Cells Due to Induction of Oxidative Stress. *Chemotherapy*. 59(3): 214-24, 2013.

Feng, Z., Hu, W., Hu, Y., and Tang, M. Acrolein is a Major Cigarette-Related Lung Cancer Agent: Preferential Binding at p53 Mutational Hotspots and Inhibition of DNA Repair. *PNAS* 10(43): 15404-15409, 2006.

Fay, MP., Freedman, LS., Clifford, CK., and Midthune, DN. Effect of Different Types and Amounts of Fat on the Development of Mammary Tumors in Rodents: A Review. *Cancer Res.* 1997 57(18): 3979-88, 1997.

Field, C. and Schley, PD. Evidence for Potential Mechanisms for the Effect of Conjugated Linoleic Acid on Tumor Metabolism and Immune Function: Lessons from n-3 Fatty Acids. *Am J Clin Nutr.* 79: 1190S-8S, 2004.

Ford, JH. Saturated Fatty Acid Metabolism is Key Link Between Cell Division, Cancer, and Senescence in Cellular and Whole Organism Aging. *AGE.* 32: 231-237, 2010.

Gago-Dominguez, M., Yuan, JM., Sun, CL., Lee, HP.,2 and Yu, MC., Opposing Effects of Dietary n-3 and n-6 Fatty acids on Mammary Carcinogenesis: The Singapore Chinese Health Study. *Brit J Cancer.* 89, 1686-1692, 2003.

Gerson, AR., Brown, JC., Thomas, R., Bernards, MA., and Staples, JF. Effects of Dietary Polyunsaturated Fatty Acids on Mitochondrial Metabolism in Mammalian Hibernation. *J Exp Biol.* 211(Pt 16): 2689-99, 2008.

Giros, A., Grzybowski, M., Sohn, VR., Pons, E., Fernandez-Morales, J., Xicola, RM., Sethi, P., Grzybowski, J,. Goel, A., Boland, CR., Gassull, MA, and Llor, X. Regulation of Colorectal Cancer Cell Apoptosis by the n-3 Polyunsaturated Fatty Acids Docosahexaenoic and Eicosapentaenoic. *Cancer Prev Res.* (Phila). 2(8): 732-42, 2009.

Gu, Z., Suburu, J., Chen, H., and Chen, YQ. Mechanisms

of Omega-3 Polyunsaturated Fatty Acids in Prostate Cancer Prevention. *Biomed Res Int*. 2013: 824563, 2013.

Guéraud, F., Taché, S., Steghens, JP., Milkovic, L., Borovic-Sunjic, S., Zarkovic, N., Gaultier, E., Naud, N., Héliès-Toussaint, C., Pierre, F., and Priymenko, N. Dietary Polyunsaturated Fatty Acids and Heme Iron Induce Oxidative Stress Biomarkers and a Cancer Promoting Environment in the Colon of Rats. *Free Radic Biol Med*. 83: 192-200, 2015.

Haines, TH. A new look at Cardiolipin. *Biochimica et Biophysica Acta*. 1788, 2009.

Hardy, S., El-Assaad, W., Przybytkowski, E., Joly, E., Prentki, M., and Langelier, Y. Saturated Fatty Acid-induced Apoptosis in MDA-MB-231 Breast Cancer Cells. A Role for Cardiolipin. *J Biol Chem*. 22;278(34):31861-70, 2003.

Hendrickse, CW., Kelly, RW., Radley, S., Donovan, IA., Keighley, MR., and Neoptolemos, JP. Lipid Peroxidation and Prostaglandins in Colorectal Cancer. *Br J Surg*. 81(8): 1219-23, 1994.

Hjelle, JJ., Grubbs, JH., and Petersen, DR. Inhibition of Mitochondrial Aldehyde Dehydrogenase by Malondialdehyde. *Toxicology Letters* (Impact Factor: 3.26). 14(1-2):35-43, 1982.

Huang, C. and Freter, C. Lipid Metabolism, Apoptosis and Cancer Therapy. *Int J Mol Sci*. 16: 924-949, 2015.

Huang, Z., Jiang, J., Tyurin, VA., Zhao, Q., Mnuskin, A.,

Ren, J., Belikova, NA., Feng, W., Kurnikov, IV., and Kagan, VE. Cardiolipin Deficiency Leads to Decreased Cardiolipin Peroxidation and Increased Resistance of Cells to Apoptosis. *Free Radic Biol Med*. 1;44(11): 1935-44, 2008.

Jung, KC., Park, CH., Hwang, YH., Rhee, HS., Lee, JH., Kim, HK., and Yang, CH. Fatty acids, Inhibitors for the DNA Binding of c-Myc/Max Dimer, Suppress Proliferation and Induce Apoptosis of Differentiated HL-60 Human Leukemia Cell. *Leukemia*. 20(1): 122-7, 2006.

Karmali, RA., Doshi, RU., Adams, L., and Choi, K. Effect of n-3 Fatty Acids on Mammary Tumorigenesis. *Adv Prostaglandin Thromboxane Leukot Res*. 17B: 886-9, 1987.

Kiebish, MA., Han, X., Cheng, H., Chuang, JH., and Seyfried, TN. Cardiolipin and Electron Transport Chain Abnormalities in Mouse Brain Tumor Mitochondria: Lipidomic Evidence Supporting the Warburg Theory of Cancer. *J Lipid Res*. 49(12): 2545-56, 2008.

Kinoshita, Y., Yoshizawa, K., Hamazaki, K., Emoto, Y., Yuri, T., Yuki, M., Shikata, N., Kawashima, H., and Tsubura, A. Mead Acid Inhibits the Growth of KPL-1 Human Breast Cancer Cells in vitro and in vivo. *Oncol Rep*. 32(4): 1385-94, 2014.

Ko, Y., Cheng, S., Lee, C., Huang, J., Huang, M., Kao, H., and Lin, H. Chinese Food Cooking and Lung Cancer in Women Nonsmokers. *Am J Epidemiol*. 151: 140-7, 2000.

Koh, WP., Dan, YY., Goh, GB., Jin, A., Wang, R., and

Yuan, JM. Dietary Fatty Acids and Risk of Hepatocellular Carcinoma in the Singapore Chinese Health Study. *Liver Int*. 36(6): 893-901, 2016.

Kramer, JK., Cruz-Hernandez, C., Deng, Z., Zhou, J., Jahreis, G., and Dugan, ME. Analysis of Conjugated Linoleic Acid and trans 18:1 Isomers in Synthetic and Animal Products. *Am J Clin Nutr*. 79(6 Suppl): 1137S-1145S, 2004.

Kroemer, G. Mitochondria in Cancer. *Oncogene*. 25: 4630-4632, 2006.

Lee, H., Wang, H., Weng, M., Hu, Y., Chen, W., Chou, D., Liu, Y., Donin, N., Huang, W.C., Lepor, H., Wu, X., Wang, H., Frederick A. Beland, F.A., and Tang, M. Acrolein- and 4-Aminobiphenyl-DNA Adducts in Human Bladder Mucosa and Tumor Tissue and Their Mutagenicity in Human Urothelial Cells. *Oncotarget*. 5(11), 2014.

Li, L., Connelly, MC., Wetmore, C., Curran, T., and Morgan, JI. Mouse Embryos Cloned from Brain Tumors. *Cancer Res*. 63(11): 2733-6, 2003.

Lowe, SW. and Lin, SW. Apoptosis in Cancer. *Carcinogenesis*. 21(3); 485-495, 2000.

Mei, S., Ni, H., Manley, S., Bockus, A., Kassel, KM., Luyendyk, JP., Copple, BL., and Ding, W. Differential Roles of Unsaturated and Saturated Fatty Acids on Autophagy and Apoptosis in Hepatocytes. *JPET*. 339: 487-498, 2011.

Macotpet, A., Suksawat, F., Sukon, P., Pimpakdee, K.,

Pattarapanwichien, E., Tangrassameeprasert, R., and Boonsiri, P. Meng, H., Shen, Y., Shen, J., Zhou, F., Shen, S., and Das, UN. Effect of n-3 and n-6 Unsaturated Fatty Acids on Prostate Cancer (PC-3) and Prostate Epithelial (RWPE-1) Cells in-vitro. *Lipids Health*. 12: 160, 2013.

Mintz, B., Illmensee, K. Normal Genetically Mosaic Mice Produced from Malignant Teratocarcinoma Cells. *Proc Natl Acad Sci* . 72(9): 3585-9, 1975.

Nicastro, HL. and Dunn, BK. Selenium and Prostate Cancer Prevention: Insights from the Selenium and Vitamin E Cancer Prevention Trial (SELECT). Nutrients. 5(4): 1122-48, 2013.

Paradies, G., Paradies, V., De Benedictis, V., Ruggiero, FM., and Petrosillo, G. Functional Role of Cardiolipin in Mitochondrial Bioenergetics. *Biochim Biophys Acta*. 1837(4): 408-17, 2014.

Qi, M., Chen, D., Liu, K., and Auborn, KJ. *n*-6 Polyunsaturated Fatty Acids Increase Skin but not Cervical Cancer in Human Papillomavirus 16 Transgenic Mice. *Cancer Research*. 62: 433-436, 2002.

Rohr-Udilova, NV., Stolze, K., Sagmeister, S., Nohl, H., Schulte-Hermann, R. and Grasl-Kraupp, B. Lipid Hydroperoxides from Processed Dietary Oils Enhance Growth of Hepatocarcinoma Cells. *Mol Nutrition & Food Res*. 52(3): 352-359, 2008.

Romero, A., Bastida, S., and Sanchez-Muniz, FJ. Cyclic Fatty Acid Monomer Formation in Domestic Frying of Frozen Foods in Sunflower Oil and High Oleic Acid

Sunflower Oil without Oil Replenishment. *Food Chem Toxicol.* 44(10): 1674-81, 2006.

Rose, G., Blackburn, H., Keys, A., Taylor, HL., Kannel, WB., Paul, O., Reid, DD., and Stamler, J. Colon Cancer and Blood and Blood-Cholesterol. *Lancet.* 303(7850): 181-183, 1974.

Rothwell, PM., Fowkes, FG., Belch, JF., Ogawa, H., Warlow, CP., and Meade, TW. Effect of Daily Aspirin on Long-term Risk of Death due to Cancer: Analysis of Individual Patient Data from Randomised Trials. *Lancet.* 377(9759): 31-41, 2011.

Ruggieri, S., Fallani, A., and Tombaccini, D. Effect of Essential Fatty Acid Deficiency on the Lipid Composition of the Yoshida Ascites Hepatoma (AH 130) and of the Liver and Blood Plasma from Host and Normal Rats. *J Lipid Res.* 17(5): 456-66, 1976.

Samhan, AK.,_Arias, Tyurina, YY., and Kagan, VE. Lipid Antioxidants: Free Radical Scavenging Versus Regulation of Enzymatic Lipid Peroxidation. *J Clin Biochem Nutr.* 48(1): 91-95, 2011.

Sapandowski, A., Stope, M., Evert, M., Zimmermann, U., Peter, D., Page, I., Burchardt, M., and Schild, L. Cardiolipin Composition Correlates with Prostate Cancer Cell Proliferation. *Mol and cell biochem.* 1, 2015.

Sasaki, T., Kobayashi, Y., Shimizu, J., Wada, M., In'nami, S., Kanke, Y., Takita, T. Effects of Dietary n-3-to-n-6 Polyunsaturated Fatty Acid Ratio on Mammary Carcinogenesis in Rats. *Nutr Cancer.* 30(2): 137-43, 1998.

Schlame, M and Ren, M. The Role of Cardiolipin in the Structural Organization of Mitochondrial Membranes. *Biochim Biophys Acta*. 1788(10): 2080-2083, 2009.

Schulze-Osthoff, K., Ferrari. F., Los. M., Wesselborg. S., and Peter, ME. Apoptosis Signaling by Death Receptors. *Eur J Biochem*. 254: 4392459, 1998.

Schumacher, MC., Laven, B., Petersson, F., Cederholm, T., Onelöv, E., Ekman, P., and Brendler, C. A Comparative Study of Tissue ω-6 and ω-3 Polyunsaturated Fatty Acids (PUFA) in Benign and Malignant Pathologic Stage pT2a Radical Prostatectomy Specimens. *Urol Oncol*. 31(3):v318-24, 2013.

Seow, A., Poh, WT., Teh, M., Eng, P., Wang, YT., Tan, WC., Yu, MC., and Lee, HP. Fumes from Meat Cooking and Lung Cancer Risk in Chinese Women. *Cancer Epidemiol Biomarkers Prev*. 9(11): 1215-21, 2000.

Shields, PG., Xu, GX., Blot, WJ., Fraumeni, JF., Trivers, GE., Pellizzari, ED., Qu, YH., Gao, YT., Harris, CC. Mutagens from Heated Chinese and U.S. Cooking Oils. *J Natl Cancer Inst*. 87(11): 836-41, 1995.

Sjaastad, AK. and Svendsen, K. Exposure to Mutagenic Aldehydes and Particulate Matter During Panfrying of Beefsteak with Margarine, Rapeseed Oil, Olive Oil or Soybean Oil. *Ann Occup Hyg*. 52(8): 739-745, 2008.

Sonestedt, E., Ericson, U., Gullberg, B., Skog, K., Olsson, HK., and Wirfalt, E. Do Both Heterocyclic Amines and Omega-6 Polyunsaturated Fatty Acids Contribute to the Incidence of Breast Cancer in Postmenopausal Women of the Malmo Diet and Cancer Cohort? *Int J Cancer*. 123: 1637-1643, 2008.

Srivastava, S., Singh, M., George, J., Bhui, K., and Shukla, Y. Genotoxic and Carcinogenic Risks Associated with the Consumption of Repeatedly Boiled Sunflower Oil. *J Agric Food Chem*. 58(20): 11179-86, 2010.

Stott-Miller, M., Neuhouser, ML., and. Stanford, JL. Consumption of Deep-fried Foods and Risk of Prostate Cancer. *Prostate*. 73(9): 960–969, 2013.

William C. Stanley, WC., Khairallah, RJ., and Dabkowski, ER. Update on Lipids and Mitochondrial Function: Impact of Dietary n-3 Polyunsaturated Fatty Acids. *Curr Opin Clin Nutr Metab Care*. 15(2): 122-126, 2012.

Stephenson, JA., Al-Taan, O., Arshad, A., Morgan, B., Metcalfe, MS., and Dennison, AR. The Multifaceted Effects of Omega-3 Polyunsaturated Fatty Acids on the Hallmarks of Cancer. *J Lipids*. 2013: 261247, 2013.

Tang, Y., Chen, Y., Jiang, H., and Nie, D. Short-chain Fatty Acids Induced Autophagy Serves as an Adaptive Strategy for Retarding Mitochondria-mediated Apoptotic Cell Death. *Cell Death and Differentiation*. 18: 602-618, 2011.

Tokudome, S., Ando, R., Ichikawa, Y., Ichikawa, H., Imaeda, N., Goto, C., Tokudome, Y., and Okuyama, H. Plasma Phospholipid Fatty Acids and Prostate Cancer Risk in the SELECT Trial. *J Natl Cancer Inst*. 105: 1132-1141, 2013.

Tomar, RS., Tsai, FC., and Sandy, MS. Evidence on the

Carcinogenicity of 3-Monochloropropane-1,2-diol (3-MCPD; α-Chlorohydrin). *OEHHA*, 2010.

Veierod, MB., Thelle, DS., and Laake, P. Diet and Risk of Cutaneous Malignant Melanoma: A Prospective Study of 50,757 Norwegian Men and Women. *Int J Cancer*. 71: 600-604, 1997.

Wang, H., Hu, Y., Tong, D., Huang, J., Gu, L., Wu, X., Chung, F., Li, G., and Tand, M. Effect of Carcinogenic Acrolein on DNA Repair and Mutagenic Susceptibility. *J Biol Chem*. 287(15): 12379-86, 2012.

Watkins, SM., Carter, LC., and German, JB. Docosahexaenoic Acid Accumulates in Cardiolipin and Enhances HT-29 Cell Oxidant Production. *J Lipid Res*. 39: 1583-1588, 1998.

Wei, Y., Dong Wang, D., Topczewski, F., and Pagliassotti, MJ. Saturated Fatty Acids Induce Endoplasmic Reticulum Stress and Apoptosis

Independently of Ceramide in Liver Cells. *Am J Physiol Endocrinol Metab*. 291: E275-E281, 2006.

Chapter 6: Immune Suppression and Inflammation

Awada, M., Soulage, CO., Meynier, A., Debard, C., Plaisancié,P., Benoit, B., Picard, G., Loizon, E., Chauvin, MA., Estienne, M., Peretti, N., Guichardant, M., Lagarde, M., Genot, C., and Michalski, MC. Dietary Oxidized n-3 PUFA Induce Oxidative Stress and Inflammation: Role of Intestinal Absorption of 4-HHE and Reactivity in Intestinal Cells. *J Lipid Res*. 53(10): 2069-80,

2012.

Calder, PC. N-3 Polyunsaturated Fatty Acids, Inflammation, and Inflammatory Diseases. *Am J Clin Nutr.* 83(suppl): 1505S-19S, 2006.

Calder, PC. Polyunsaturated Fatty Acids and Inflammatory Processes: New Twists in an Old Tale. *Biochimie.* 91: 791-795, 2009.

Calder, PC. Long-chain Polyunsaturated Fatty Acids and Inflammation. *Scandinavian Journal of Food and Nutrition.* 50(S2): 54-61, 2006.

Calder, PC. Omega-3 Fatty Acids and Inflammatory Processes. *Nutrients.* 2: 355-374, 2010.

Calder, PC. and Grimble, RF. Polyunsaturated Fatty Acids, Inflammation and Immunity. *European Journal of Clinical Nutrition.* 56(Suppl 3): S14-S19, 2002.

Cao, W., Ramakrishnan, R., Tyurin, VA., Veglia ,F., Condamine, T., Amoscato, A., Mohammadyani, D., Johnson, JJ., Zhang, LM., Klein-Seetharaman, J., Celis, E., Kagan, VE., and Gabrilovich, DI. Oxidized Lipids Block Antigen Cross-presentation by Dendritic Cells in Cancer. *J Immunol.* 192(6): 2920-31, 2014.

Cleland, LG., Gibson, RA., Neumann, MA., Hamazaki, T., Akimoto, K., and James, MJ. Dietary (n-9) Eicosatrienoic Acid from a Cultured Fungus Inhibits Leukotriene B4 Synthesis in Rats and the Effect is Modified by Dietary Linoleic Acid. *J Nutr.* 126(6): 1534-40 1996.

Cleland, LG., James, MJ., Neumann, MA., D'Angelo, M., Gibson, RA. Linoleate Inhibits EPA Incorporation from

Dietary Fish-oil Supplements in Human Subjects. *Am J Clin Nutr*. 55(2): 395-9, 1992.

Cunningham-Rundles, S. Is the Fatty Acid Composition of Immune Cells the Key to Normal Variations in Human Immune Response? *Am J Clin Nutr*. 77: 1096-7, 2003.

Curiel, TJ. Regulatory T Cells and Treatment of Cancer. *Curr Opin Immunol*. 20(2): 241-246, 2008.

Eiró, N. and Vizoso, FJ. Inflammation and Cancer. *World J Gastrointest Surg*. 4(3): 62-72, 2012.

Forman, BM., Chen, J., and Evans, RM. Hypolipidemic Drugs, Polyunsaturated Fatty Acids, and Eicosanoids are Ligands for Peroxisome Proliferator-activated Receptors α and δ. *Proc. Natl. Acad. Sci*. 94: 4312-4317, 1997.

Grimble, RF. and Tappia, PS. Modulation of Pro-inflammatory Cytokine Biology by Unsaturated Fatty Acids. *Z Ernahrungswiss*. 37 Suppl 1:57, 1998.

Grivennikov, SI., Greten, FR., and Karin, M. Immunity, Inflammation, and Cancer. *Cell*. 140(6): 883-899, 2010.

Gruber, F., Ornelas, CM., Karner, S., Narzt, MS., Nagelreiter, IM., Gschwandtner, M., Bochkov, V., and Tschachler. E. Nrf2 Deficiency Causes Lipid Oxidation, Inflammation, and Matrix-Protease Expression in DHA-Supplemented and UVA-Irradiated Skin Fibroblasts. *Free Radic Biol Med*. 88(Pt B): 439-51, 2015.

Haberland, ME., Fless, GM., Scanu, AM., and Fogelman, AM. Malondialdehyde Modification of Lipoprotein(a)

Produces Avid Uptake by Human Monocyte-Macrophages. *J Biol Chem.* 267(6): 4143-51,1992.

Harbige, LS. Dietary n-6 and n-3 Fatty Acids in Immunity and Autoimmune Disease. *Proc Nutr Soc.* 57(4): 555-62, 1998.

Hoesel, B. and Schmid, JA. The Complexity of NF-κB Signaling in Inflammation and Cancer. *Molecular Cancer.* 12: 86, 2013.

Hsu, L., Wen, Z., Chen, H., Lin, H., Chiu, C., and Wu, H. Evaluation of the Anti-Inflammatory Activities of 5,8,11-cis-Eicosatrienoic Acid. *Food and Nutrition Sciences.* 4: 113-119, 2013.

Issazadeh-Navikas, S., Teimer, R.,and Bockermann, R. Influence of Dietary Components on Regulatory T Cells. *Mol Med.* 18: 95-110, 2012.

Jameel, F., Phang, M., Wood, LG., and Garg, ML. Acute Effects of Feeding Fructose, Glucose and Sucrose on Blood Lipid Levels and Systemic Inflammation. *Lipids Health Dis.* 13: 195, 2014.

James, MJ., Gibson, RA. and Cleland, LG. Dietary Polyunsaturated Fatty Acids and Inflammatory Mediator Production. *Am J Clin Nutr.* 71(suppl): 343S-8S, 2000.

James, MJ. Gibson, RA., Neumann, MA., and Cleland, LG. Effect of Dietary Supplementation with n-9 Eicosatrienoic Acid on Leukotriene B4 Synthesis in Rats: A Novel Approach to Inhibition of Eicosanoid Synthesis. *J Exp Med.* 178(6): 2261-5, 1993.

Karavitis, J., Hix, LM., Shi, YH., Schultz, R.F, Khazaie,

K., and Zhang, M. Regulation of COX2 Expression in Mouse Mammary Tumor Cells Controls Bone Metastasis and PGE2-Induction of Regulatory T Cell Migration. *PLoS One*. 7(9): e46342, 2012.

Kawamori, T., Uchiya, N., Sugimura, T. and Wakabayashi, K. Enhancement of Colon Carcinogenesis by Prostaglandin E2 Administration. *Proc Nutr Soc.* 57(4): 555-62, 1998.

Kim, W., Khan, NA., McMurray, DN., Prior, IA., Wang, N., and Chapkin, RS. Regulatory Activity of Polyunsaturated Fatty Acids in T-Cell Signaling. *Prog Lipid Res*. 49(3): 250-261, 2010.

Kim, W. and Lee, H. Advances in Nutritional Research on Regulatory T-Cells. *Nutrients.* 5: 4305-4315, 2013.

Kraaij, MD., Savage, ND., Van der Kooij, SW., Koekkoek, K., Wang, J., Van den Berg, JM., Ottenhoff, TH., Kuijpers, TW., Holmdahl, R., Van Kooten, C., and Gelderman, KA. Induction of Regulatory T cells by Macrophages is Dependent on Production of Reactive Oxygen Species. *Proc Natl Acad Sci*. 107(41): 17686-91, 2010.

Lefkowith, JB., Morrison, A, Lee, V., and Rogers, M. Manipulation of the Acute Inflammatory Response by Dietary Polyunsaturated Fatty Acid Modulation. *J Immunol*. 145(5): 1523-9, 1990.

Ling, PR., Malkan, A., Le, HD., Puder M., and Bistrian, BR. Arachidonic Acid and Docosahexaenoic Acid Supplemented to an Essential Fatty Acid-Deficient Diet Alters the Response to Endotoxin in Rats. *Metabolism*.

61(3): 395-406, 2013.

Lian, M., Luo, W., Sui, Y., Li, Z., and Hua, J. Dietary n-3 PUFA Protects Mice from Con A Induced Liver Injury by Modulating Regulatory T Cells and PPAR-γ Expression. *PLoS One*, 10(7), 2015.

Mahic, M., Yaqub, S., Johansson, CC., Taskén, K., and Aandahl, EM. FOXP3+CD4+CD25+ Adaptive Regulatory T Cells Express Cyclooxygenase-2 and Suppress Effector T Cells by a Prostaglandin E2-Dependent Mechanism. *J of Immunology*, 177: 246-254, 2006.

Masini, E., Palmerani, B., Gambassi, F., Pistelli, A., Giannella, E., Occupati, B., Ciuffi, M., Sacchi, TB., and Mannaioni, PF. Histamine Release from Rat Mast Cells Induced by Metabolic Activation of Polyunsaturated Fatty Acids into Free Radicals. *Biochem Pharmacol*. 39(5): 879-89, 1990.

Mougiakakos, D., Choudhury, A., Lladser, A., Kiessling, R., and Johansson, CC. Regulatory T Cells in Cancer. *Adv Cancer Res*. 107: 57-117, 2010.

Nicolaou, A., Mauro, C., Urquhart, P., and Marelli-Berg, F. Polyunsaturated Fatty Acid-derived Lipid Mediators and T Cell Function. *Front Immunol*. 5(75): 1-15, 2014.

Nizar, S., Copier, J., Meyer, B., Bodman-Smith, M., Galustian, C., Kumar, D., and Dalgleish, A. T-regulatory Cell Modulation: The Future of Cancer Immunotherapy. *Br J Cancer*. 100(11): 1697-703, 2009.

Perrin-Cocon, L., Diaz, O., André, P., and Lotteau, V. Modified Lipoproteins Provide Lipids that Modulate

Dendritic Cell Immune Function. *Biochimie*. 95(1): 103-8, 2013.

Quaschning, T., Mainka, T., Nauck, M., Rump, LC., Wanner, C., and Krämer-Guth, A. Immunosuppression Enhances Atherogenicity of Lipid Profile After Transplantation. Kidney Int Suppl. 71: S235-7, 1999.

Raghavan, S., Subramaniyam, G., and Shanmugam, N. Proinflammatory Effects of Malondialdehyde in Lymphocytes. *J Leukocyte Biol*. 92: 1055-1067, 2012.

Raphael, W. and Sordillo, LM. Dietary Polyunsaturated Fatty Acids and Inflammation: The Role of Phospholipid Biosynthesis. *Int J Mol Sci*. 14: 21167-21188, 2013.

Reeve, VE., Bosnic, M., and Boehm-Wilcox, C. Dependence of Photocarcinogenesis and Photoimmunosuppression in the Hairless Mouse on Dietary Polyunsaturated Fat. *Cancer Letters*, 108(2): 271-279, 1996.

Rothwell, PM., Wilson, M., Price, JF., Belch, JF., Meade, TW., and Mehta, Z. Effect of Daily Aspirin on Risk of Cancer Metastasis: A Study of Incident Cancers During Randomised Controlled Trials. *Lancet*. 379(9826): 1591-601, 2012.

Shaikh, SR., and Edidin, M. Polyunsaturated Fatty Acids, Membrane Organization, T cells, and Antigen Presentation. *Am J Clin Nutr*. 84: 1277-89, 2006.

Smith, AD., Conroy, DM., and Belin, J. Membrane Lipid Modification and Immune Function. *Proceedings of the Nutrition Society*, 44: 201-1985.

Sweeney, B., Puri, P., and Reen, DJ. Modulation of Immune Cell Function by Polyunsaturated Fatty Acids. *Pediatric Surgery International*. 21(5): 335-340, 2005.

Vitale, JJ. and Broitman, SA. Lipids and Immune Function. *Cancer Research*. 41: 3706-3710, 1981.

Yaqoob, P. Fatty Acids as Gatekeepers of Immune Cell Regulation. *Trends in Immunology*, 24(12), 2003.

Zaguri, R., Verbovetski, I., Atallah, M., Trahtemberg, U., Krispin, A., Nahari, E., Leitersdorf, E., and Mevorach, D. 'Danger' Effect of Low-Density Lipoprotein (LDL) and Oxidized LDL on Human Immature Dendritic Cells. *Clin Exp Immunol*. 149(3): 543-52, 2007.

Chapter 7: Obesity and Diabetes

Ahmad, R., Al-Mass, A., Atizado, V., Al-Hubail, A., Al-Ghimlas, F., Al-Arouj, M., Bennakhi, A., Dermime, S., Behbehani, K. Elevated Expression of the Toll like Receptors 2 and 4 in Obese Individuals: Its Significance for Obesity-induced Inflammation. *J Inflamm (Lond)*. 9(1): 48, 2012.

Amini, P., Wadden, D., Cahill, F., Randell, E., Vasdev, S., Chen, X., Gulliver, W., Zhang, W., Zhang, H., Yi, Y., and Sun, G. Serum Acylated Ghrelin is Negatively Correlated with the Insulin Resistance in the CODING Study. *PLoS One*. 7(9): e45657, 2012.

Anson, RM., Guo, Z., de Cabo, R., Iyun, T., Rios, M., Hagepanos, A., Ingram, DK., Lane, MA., Mattson, MP. Intermittent Fasting Dissociates Beneficial Effects of Dietary Restriction on Glucose Metabolism and Neuronal

Resistance to Injury from Calorie Intake. *Proc Natl Acad Sci*. 100(10): 6216-20, 2003.

Anderwald, CH., Tura, A., Gessl, A., Smajis, S., Bieglmayer, C., Marculescu, R., Luger, A., Pacini, G., and Krebs, M. Whole-Body Insulin Sensitivity Rather than Body-Mass-Index Determines Fasting and Post-Glucose-Load Growth Hormone Concentrations. *PLoS One*. 9(12):e115184, 2014.

Anson, RM., Guo, Z., de Cabo, R., Iyun, T., Rios, M., Hagepanos, A., Ingram, DK., Lane, MA., and Mattson, MP. Intermittent Fasting Dissociates Beneficial Effects of Dietary Restriction on Glucose Metabolism and Neuronal Resistance to Injury from Calorie Intake. *Proc Natl Acad Sci*. 100(10): 6216-20, 2003.

Barnard, RJ., Roberts, CK., Varon, SM., and Berger, JJ. Diet-induced Insulin Resistance Precedes Other Aspects of the Metabolic Syndrome. *J Appl Physiol*. 84(4): 1311-5, 1998 .

Basciano, H., Federico, L. and Adeli, K. Fructose, Insulin Resistance, and Metabolic Dyslipidemia. *Nutrition & Metabolism*. 2:5, 2005.

Batterham, RL., Cohen, MA., Ellis, SM., Le Roux, CW., Withers, DJ., Frost, GS., Ghatei, MA., and Bloom, SR. Inhibition of Food Intake in Obese Subjects by Peptide YY_{3-36}. *N Engl J Med* 349: 941-8, 2003.

Berryman, DE., List, EO., Sackmann-Sala, L., Lubbers, E., Munn, R., Kopchick, JJ. Growth Hormone and Adipose Tissue: Beyond the Adipocyte. *Growth Horm IGF*

Res. (3):113-23, 2011.

Blackard, WG., Hull, EW., and Lopez, A. Effect of Lipids on Growth Hormone Secretion in Humans. *J Clin Invest.* 50(7): 1439-43, 1971.

Bokarewa, M., Nagaev, I., Dahlberg, L., Smith, U., and Tarkowski, A. Resistin, an Adipokine with Potent Pro-inflammatory Properties. *J Immunology,* 174: 5789–5795, 2005.

Burghardt, PR., Kemmerer, ES., Buck, BJ., Osetek, AJ., Yan, C., Koch, LG., Britton, SL., Evans, SJ. Dietary n-3:n-6 Fatty Acid Ratios Differentially Influence Hormonal Signature in a Rodent Model of Metabolic Syndrome Relative to Healthy Controls. *Nutr Metab (Lond).* 7:53, 2010.

Cammisotto, PG., Gelinas, Y., Deshaies, Y., and Buko-wiecki, LJ. Regulation of Leptin Secretion from White Adipocytes by Free Fatty Acids. *Am J Physiol Endocrinol Metab.* 285: E521–E526, 2003.

Carr, RD., Larsen, MO., Winzell, MS., Jelic, K., Lindgren, O., Deacon, CF., and Ahrén, B. Incretin and islet hormo-nal responses to fat and protein ingestion in healthy men. *Am J Physiol Endocrinol Metab.* 295(4): E779-84, 2008.

Castro-Webb, N., Ruiz-Narváez, EA., and Campos, H. Cross-sectional Study of Conjugated Linoleic Acid in Adipose Tissue and Risk of Diabetes. *Am J Clin Nutr.* 96(1):175-81, 2012.

Cernea, S and Dobreanu,M. Diabetes and Beta Cell

Function: From Mechanisms to Evaluation and Clinical Implications. *Biochemia Medica* 23(3): 266-80, 2013.

Cheng, L., Yu, Y., Zhang, Q., Szabo, A., Wang, H., Huang, XF. Arachidonic Acid Impairs Hypothalamic Leptin Signaling and Hepatic Energy Homeostasis in Mice. *Mol Cell Endocrinol*. 412: 12-8, 2015.

Collier, G. and O'Dea, K. The Effect of Coingestion of Fat on the Glucose, Insulin, and Gastric Inhibitory Polypeptide Responses to Carbohydrate and Protein. *Am J Clin Nutr*. 37(6): 941-4, 1983.

de Ferranti, S. and Mozaffarian, D. The Perfect Storm: Obesity, Adipocyte Dysfunction, and Metabolic Consequences. *Clin Chem*. 54(6): 945–955, 2008.

Deol, P., Evans, JR., Dhahbi, J., Chellappa, K., Han, DS., Spindler, S., Sladek, FM. Soybean Oil Is More Obesogenic and Diabetogenic than Coconut Oil and Fructose in Mouse: Potential Role for the Liver. *PLoS One*. 10(7): e0132672, 2015.

Dulloo, AG., Gubler, M., Montani, JP., Seydoux, J., and Solinas, G. Substrate Cycling Between de novo Lipogenesis and Lipid Oxidation: A Thermogenic Mechanism Against Skeletal Muscle Lipotoxicity and Glucolipotoxicity. Int J Obes Relat Metab Disord. 28 Suppl 4: S29-37, 2004.

Eitel, K., Staiger, H., Brendel, MD., Brandhorst, D., Bretzel, RG., Häring, HU., and Kellerer, M. Different Role of Saturated and Unsaturated Fatty Acids in Beta-cell Apoptosis. *Biochem Biophys Res Commun*. 299(5): 853-6,

2002.

Ercan, S., Kencebay, C., Basaranlar, G., Ozcan, F., Derin, N., Aslan, M. Induction of Omega 6 Inflammatory Pathway by Sodium Metabisulfite in Rat Liver and its Attenuation by Ghrelin. *Lipids Health Dis*. 14:7, 2015.

Fan, C. Liu, X., Shen, W., Deckelbaum, RJ., and Qi, K. The Regulation of Leptin, Leptin Receptor and Pro-opiomelanocortin Expression by N-3 PUFAs in Diet-Induced Obese Mice Is Not Related to the Methylation of Their Promoters. *Nutrition & Metabolism*. 8:31, 2011.

Frangioudakis, G., Garrard, J., Raddatz, K., Nadler, JL., Mitchell, TW., and Schmitz-Peiffer, C. Saturated- and n-6 Polyunsaturated-Fat Diets Each Induce Ceramide Accumulation in Mouse Skeletal Muscle: Reversal and Improvement of Glucose Tolerance by Lipid Metabolism Inhibitors. *Endocrinology*. 151(9): 4187-4196, 2010.

Furukawa, S., Fujita, T., Shimabukuro, M., Iwaki, M., Yamada, Y., Nakajima, Y, Nakayama, O., Makishima, M., Matsuda, M., Shimomura, I. Increased Oxidative Stress in Obesity and its Impact on Metabolic Syndrome. *J Clin Invest*. 114(12): 1752-61, 2004.

Glauber, H., Wallace, P., Griver, K., and Brechtel, G. Adverse Metabolic Effect of Omega-3 Fatty Acids in Non-Insulin-Dependent Diabetes Mellitus. *Ann Intern Med*. 108(5): 663-668, 1988.

Ho, KY., Veldhuis, JD., Johnson, ML., Furlanetto, R., Evans, WS., Alberti, KG., Thorner, MO. Fasting Enhances Growth Hormone Secretion and Amplifies the Complex Rhythms of Growth Hormone Secretion in Man. *J Clin*

Invest. 81(4):968-75, 1988.

Hurt, RT., Frazier, TH., Matheson, PJ., Cave, MC., Garrison, RN., McClain, CJ., and McClave, SA. Obesity and Inflammation: Should the Principles of Immunonutrition Be Applied to This Disease Process? *Curr Gastroenterol Rep.* 9(4):305-6, 2007.

Jump, DB. Fatty Acid Regulation of Hepatic Lipid Metabolism. *Curr Opin Clin Nutr Metab Care.* 14(2): 115–120, 2011.

Karra, E., Chandarana, K., and Batterham, RL. The role of Peptide YY in Appetite Regulation and Obesity. *J Physiol.* 587(1): 19–25, 2009.

Karlström, BE., Järvi, AE., Byberg, L., Berglund, LG., and Vessby, BO. Fatty Fish in the Diet of Patients with Type 2 Diabetes: Comparison of the Metabolic Effects of Foods Rich in n-3 and n-6 Fatty Acids. *Am J Clin Nutr.* 94: 26–33, 2011.

Kim, SJ., Choi, Y., Choi, YH., and Park, T. Obesity Activates Toll-like Receptor-mediated Proinflammatory Signaling Cascades in the Adipose Tissue of Mice. *J Nutr Biochem.* 23(2): 113-22, 2012.

Kim, W. and Egan, JM. The Role of Incretins in Glucose Homeostasis and Diabetes Treatment. *Pharmacol Rev.* 60(4): 470–512, 2008.

Kojima, M., Hosoda, H., Date, Y., Nakazato, M., Matsuo, H., and Kangawa, K. Ghrelin is a Growth-hormone-releasing Acylated Peptide from Stomach. *Nature.*

402(6762): 656-60, 1999.

Koliaki, C., Kokkinos, A., Tentolouris, N., and Katsilambros, N. The Effect of Ingested Macronutrients on Postprandial Ghrelin Response: A Critical Review of Existing Literature Data. *Int J Pept*. 2010. pii: 710852, 2010.

Korotkova, M., Gabrielsson, B., Lönn, M., Hanson, LA., Strandvik, B. Leptin Levels in Rat Offspring are Modified by the Ratio of Linoleic to alpha-linolenic Acid in the Maternal Diet. *J Lipid Res*. 2002 Oct;43(10):1743-9.

Kozimor, A., Chang, H., and Cooper, JA. Effects of Dietary Fatty Acid Composition from a High Fat Meal on Satiety. *Appetite* 69: 39–45, 2013.

Kratz, M., Swarbrick, MM., Callahan, HS., Matthys, CC., Havel, PJ., Weigle, DS. Effect of Dietary n-3 Polyunsaturated Fatty Acids on Plasma Total and High-molecular-weight Adiponectin Concentrations in Overweight to Moderately Obese Men and Women. *Am J Clin Nutr*. 87(2): 347-53, 2008.

Lee, SM., Cho, YH., Lee, SY., Jeong, DW., Cho, AR., Jeon, JS., Park, EJ., Kim, YJ., Lee, JG., Yi, YH., Tak, YJ., Hwang, HR., Lee, SH., Han, J. Urinary Malondialdehyde Is Associated with Visceral Abdominal Obesity in Middle-Aged Men. *Mediators Inflamm*. 2015: 524291, 2015.

Lihn, AS., Pedersen, SB., Richelsen, B. Adiponectin: Action, Regulation and Association to Insulin Sensitivity. *Obes Rev*. 6(1):13-21, 2005.

Lumeng, CN. and Saltiel, AR. Inflammatory Links between Obesity and Metabolic Disease. *J Clin Invest.* 121(6):2111–2117, 2011.

Ley, RE. Obesity and the Human Microbiome. *Curr Opin Gastroentrtol.* 26(1): 5-11, 2010.

Liu, HQ., Qiu, Y., Mu, Y., Zhang, XJ., Liu, L., Hou, XH., Zhang, L., Xu, XN., Ji, AL., Cao, R., Yang. RH, and Wang, F. A High Ratio of Dietary n-3/n-6 Polyunsaturated Fatty Acids Improves Obesity-linked Inflammation and Insulin Resistance Through Suppressing Activation of TLR4 in SD Rats. *Nutr Res.* 33(10): 849-58, 2013.

Martınez-Victoria, E. and Yago, MD. Omega 3 Polyunsaturated Fatty Acids and Body Weight. *Brit J of Nutr.* 107:S107–S116, 2012.

Mattson, MP. Roles of the Lipid Peroxidation Product 4-Hydroxynonenal in Obesity, the Metabolic Syndrome, and Associated Vascular and Neurodegenerative Disorders. *Exp Gerontol.* 44(10): 625–633, 2009.

Miccoli, R., Bianchi, C., Penno, G., and Del Prato, S. Insulin Resistance and Lipid Disorders. *Future Lipidology.* 3(6):651-664, 2008.

Misra, A., Singhal, N., and Khurana, L. Obesity, the Metabolic Syndrome, and Type 2 Diabetes in Developing Countries: Role of Dietary Fats and Oils. *J Am Coll Nutr.* 29(3 Suppl): 289S-301S, 2010.

Moreto, F., de Oliveira, EP., Manda, RM., Burini, RC. The Higher Plasma Malondialdehyde Concentrations

Are Determined by Metabolic Syndrome-Related Glu-colipotoxicity. *Oxid Med Cell Longev*. 2014:505368, 2014.

Mostowik, M., Gajos, G., Zalewski, J., Nessler, J., Undas, A. Omega-3 Polyunsaturated Fatty Acids Increase Plasma Adiponectin to Leptin Ratio in Stable Coronary Artery Disease. *Cardiovasc Drugs Ther*. 27(4): 289-95, 2013.

Nass, RM., Gaylinn, BD., Rogol, AD., and Thorner, MO. Ghrelin and Growth Hormone: Story in Reverse. *Proc Natl Acad Sci*. 107(19): 8501-2, 2010.

Nuernberg, K., Breier, BH., Jayasinghe, SN., Bergmann, H., Thompson, N., Nuernberg, G., Dannenberger, D., Schneider, F., Renne, U., Langhammer, M., Huber, K. Metabolic Responses to High-fat Diets Rich in n-3 or n-6 Long-chain Polyunsaturated Fatty Acids in Mice Selected for Either High Body Weight or Leanness Explain Different Health Outcomes. *Nutr Metab (Lond)*. 8(1):56, 2011.

Nuttall, FQ. and Gannon, MC. Dietary Protein and the Blood Glucose Concentration. *Diabetes*. 62: 1371-1372, 2013.

Pereira, S., Breen, DM., Naassan, AE., Wang, PY., Uchino, H., Fantus, IG., Carpentier, AC., Gutierrez-Juarez, R., Brindley DN., Lam, TK., and Giacca, A. In Vivo Effects of Polyunsaturated, Monounsaturated, and Saturated Fatty Acids on Hepatic and Peripheral Insulin Sensitivity. *Metabolism*. 64(2): 315-22, 2015.

Phillips, CM., Goumidi, L., Bertrais, S., Field, MR., Ordovas, JM., Cupples, LA., Defoort, C., Lovegrove, JA.,

Drevon, CA., Blaak, EE., Gibney, MJ., Kiec-Wilk, B., Karlstrom, B., Lopez-Miranda. J., McManus, R., Hercberg, S., Lairon, D., Planells, R., Roche, HM. Leptin Receptor Polymorphisms Interact with Polyunsaturated Fatty Acids to Augment Risk of Insulin Resistance and Metabolic Syndrome in Adults. *J Nutr.* 140(2):238-44, 2010.

Roden, M., Price, TB., Perseghin, G., Petersen, KF., Rothman, DL., Cline, GW., and Shulman, GI. Mechanism of Free Fatty Acid-induced Insulin Resistance in Humans. *J Clin Invest.* 97(12): 2859-65, 1996.

Rodríguez-Hernández, H., Simental-Mendía, LE., Rodríguez-Ramírez, G., and Reyes-Romero, MA. Obesity and Inflammation: Epidemiology, Risk Factors, and Markers of Inflammation. *Int J Endocrinol.* 2013:678159, 2013.

Rudling, M., Norstedt, G., Olivecrona, H., Reihnér, E., Gustafsson, JA., and Angelin, B. Importance of growth hormone for the induction of hepatic low density lipoprotein receptors. Proc Natl Acad Sci. 89(15): 6983-7, 1992.

Sankhla, M., Sharma, TK., Mathur, K., Rathor, JS., Butolia, V., Gadhok, AK., Vardey, SK., Sinha, M., Kaushik, GG. Relationship of oxidative stress with obesity and its role in obesity induced metabolic syndrome. *Clin Lab.* 58(5-6): 385-92, 2012.

Shah, M., Adams-Huet, B., Brinkley, L., Grundy, SM., and Garg, A. Lipid, Glycemic, and Insulin Responses to

Meals Rich in Saturated, cis-Monounsaturated, and Polyunsaturated (n-3 and n-6) Fatty Acids in Subjects with Type 2 Diabetes. *Diabetes Care*. (12): 2993-8 2007.

Sivitz, WI. Mitochondrial Dysfunction in Obesity and Diabetes. *US Endocrinology*. 6:20-7, 2010.

Stienstra, R., Duval, C., Muller, M. and Kersten, S. PPARs, Obesity, and Inflammation. *PPAR Research. 2007(95974), 2007*.

Teng, KT., Chang, CY., Chang, LF., Nesaretnam, K. Modulation of Obesity-Induced Inflammation by Dietary Fats: Mechanisms and Clinical Evidence. *Nutr J*. 13: 12, 2014.

Tekeleselassie, AW., Goh, YM., Rajion,MA., Motshakeri, M., and Ebrahimi, M. A High-Fat Diet Enriched with Low Omega-6 to Omega-3 Fatty Acid Ratio Reduced Fat Cellularity and Plasma Leptin Concentration in *Sprague-Dawley* Rats. *Scientific World Journal*. 2013: 757593, 2013.

Tong, J., Prigeon, RL., Davis, HW., Bidlingmaier, M., Kahn, SE., Cummings, DE., Tschöp, MH., and D'Alessio, D. Ghrelin Suppresses Glucose-Stimulated Insulin Secretion and Deteriorates Glucose Tolerance in Healthy Humans. *Diabetes*. 59(9): 2145-51, 2010.

Trepanowski, JF. And Bloomer, RJ. The Impact of Religious Fasting on Human Health. *Nutr J*. 9: 57, 2010.

Vachharajani, V. and Granger, DN. Adipose Tissue: A Motor for the Inflammation Associated with Obesity. *IUBMB Life*. 61(4): 424–430, 2009.

van Woudenbergh, GJ., van Ballegooijen, AJ., Kuijsten,

A., Sijbrands, EJ., van Rooij, FJ., Geleijnse, JM., Hofman, A., Witteman, JC., and Feskens, EJ. Eating Fish and Risk of Type 2 Diabetes: A Population-based, Prospective Follow-up Study. *Diabetes Care*. 32(11): 2021-6, 2009.

Vanhala, M., Saltevo, J., Soininen, P., Kautiainen, H., Kangas, AJ., Ala-Korpela, M., Mäntyselkä, P. Serum Omega-6 Polyunsaturated Fatty Acids and the Metabolic Syndrome: A Longitudinal Population-based Cohort Study. *Am J Epidemiol*. 176(3): 253-60, 2012.

Vaughan, RA., Garcia-Smith, R., Bisoffi, M., Conn, CA., and Trujillo, KA. Conjugated Linoleic Acid or Omega-3 Fatty acids Increase Mitochondrial Biosynthesis and Metabolism in Skeletal Muscle Cells. *Lipids Health Dis*. 11: 142, 2012.

Vijayakumar, A., Novosyadlyy. R., Wu, Y., Yakar, S., and LeRoith, D. Biological Effects of Growth Hormone on Carbohydrate and Lipid Metabolism. *Growth Horm IGF Res*. 20(1): 1-7, 2010.

Wan, R., Ahmet, I., Brown, M., Cheng, A., Kamimura, N., Talan, M., Mattson, MP. Cardioprotective Effect of Intermittent Fasting is Associated with an Elevation of Adiponectin Levels in Rats. *J Nutr Biochem*. 21(5): 413-7, 2010.

Wang, H., Storlien, LH., and Huang, XF. Effects of Dietary Fat Types on Body Fatness, Leptin, and ARC Leptin Receptor, NPY, and AgRP mRNA Expression. Am J *Physiol Endocrinol Metab*. 282(6): E1352-9, 2002.

Wang, X. and Chan, CB. n-3 Polyunsaturated Fatty Acids and Insulin Secretion. *J Endocrinol*. 224(3): R97-106, 2015.

Wang, Z., Dou, X., Gu, D., Shen, C., Yao, T., Nguyen, V., Braunschweig, C., Song, Z. 4-Hydroxynonenal Differentially Regulates Adiponectin Gene Expression and Secretion via Activating PPARγ and Accelerating Ubiquitin–proteasome Degradation. *Mol Cell Endocrinol*. 349(2): 222-31, 2012.

Wong, CK., Botta, A., Pither, J., Dai, C., Gibson, WT., Ghosh, S. A High-fat Diet Rich in Corn Oil Reduces Spontaneous Locomotor Activity and Induces Insulin Resistance in Mice. *J Nutr Biochem*. 26(4): 319-26, 2015.

Zarrinpar, A. and Loomba, R. Review Article: The Emerging Interplay Among the Gastrointestinal Tract, Bile Acids and Incretins in the Pathogenesis of Diabetes and Non-alcoholic Fatty Liver Disease. *Aliment Pharmacol Ther*. 36(10): 909-921, 2012.

Zhang, X., Wang, Z., Li, J., Gu, D., Li, S., Shen, C., Song, Z. Increased 4-Hydroxynonenal Formation Contributes to Obesity-Related Lipolytic Activation in Adipocytes. *PLoS One*. 8(8): e70663, 2013.

Zeyda, M. and Stulnig, TM. Obesity, Inflammation, and Insulin Resistance --A Mini-Review. *Gerontology*. 55:379–386, 2009.

Chapter 8: Diet Modification

Bengtsson, BA., Brummer, RJ., Edén, S., Rosén, T., and Sjöström, L. Effects of Growth Hormone on Fat Mass and Fat Distribution. *Acta Paediatr*. Suppl. 383: 62-5; discussion 66, 1992.

Caton, PW., Nayuni, NK., Khan, NQ., Wood, EG., Corder, R. Fructose Induces Gluconeogenesis and Lipogenesis Through a SIRT1-dependent Mechanism. *J Endocrinol*. 208(3): 273-83, 2011.

Faeh, D., Minehira, K., Schwarz, JM., Periasamy, R., Park, S., Tappy, L. Effect of Fructose Overfeeding and Fish Oil Administration on Hepatic De Novo Lipogenesis and Insulin Sensitivity in Healthy Men. *Diabetes*. 54(7):1907-13, 2005.

Johannsson, G., Mårin, P., Lönn, L., Ottosson, M., Stenlöf, K., Björntorp, P., Sjöström, L., and Bengtsson, BA. Growth Hormone Treatment of Abdominally Obese Men Reduces Abdominal Fat Mass, Improves Glucose and Lipoprotein Metabolism, and Reduces Diastolic Blood Pressure. *J Clin Endocrinol Metab*. 82(3): 727-34, 1997.

Chapter 9: Dysbiosis

Alcock, J. and Lin, HC. Fatty Acids from Diet and Microbiota Regulate Energy Metabolism. *F1000Research* 4: 738, 2015.

Alcock, J., Maley, CC., and Aktipis, CA. Is Eating Behavior Manipulated by the Gastrointestinal Microbiota? Evolutionary Pressures and Potential Mechanisms. *Bioessays* 36: 940-949, 2014.

Amar, J., Lange, C., Payros, G., Garret, C., Chabo, C.,

Lantieri, O., Courtney, M., Marre, M., Charles, MA., Balkau, B., Burcelin, R; and D.E.S.I.R. Study Group. Blood Microbiota Dysbiosis Is Associated with the Onset of Cardiovascular Events in a Large General Population: The D.E.S.I.R. Study. *PLoS One.* 8(1): e54461, 2013.

Barrett, E., Fitzgerald, P., Dinan, TG., Cryan, JF., Ross, RP., Quigley, EM., Shanahan, F., Kiely, B., Fitzgerald, GF., O'Toole, PW., and Stanton, C. Bifidobacterium breve with a-Linolenic Acid and Linoleic Acid Alters Fatty Acid Metabolism in the Maternal Separation Model of Irritable Bowel Syndrome. *PLoS One.* 7(11): e48159, 2012.

Cani, PD., Amar, J., Iglesias, MA., Poggi, M., Knauf, C., Bastelica, D., Neyrinck, AM., Fava, F., Tuohy, KM., Chabo, C., Waget, A., Delmée, E., Cousin, B., Sulpice, T., Chamontin, B., Ferrières, J., Tanti, JF., Gibson, GR., Casteilla, L., Delzenne, NM., Alessi, MC., and Burcelin, R. Metabolic Endotoxemia Initiates Obesity and Insulin Resistance. *Diabetes.* 56(7):1761-72. Epub 2007.

Clark, SE. and Weiser, JN. Microbial Modulation of Host Immunity with the Small Molecule Phosphorylcholine. *Infect Immun.* 81(2): 392-401, 2013.

Denou, E., Lolmède, K., Garidou, L., Pomie, C., Chabo, C., Lau, TC., Fullerton, MD., Nigro, G., Zakaroff-Girard, A., Luche, E., Garret, C., Serino, M., Amar, J., Courtney, M., Cavallari, JF., Henriksbo, BD., Barra, NG., Foley, KP., McPhee, JB., Duggan, BM., O'Neill, HM., Lee, AJ., Sansonetti, P., Ashkar, AA., Khan, WI., Surette, MG., Bouloumié, A., Steinberg, GR., Burcelin, R., Schertzer,

JD. Defective NOD2 Peptidoglycan Sensing Promotes Diet-induced Inflammation, Dysbiosis, and Insulin Resistance. *EMBO Mol Med*. 7(3): 259-74, 2015.

Elkind, MSV. Infectious Burden: A New Risk Factor and Treatment Target for Atherosclerosis. *Infect Disord Drug Targets*. 10(2): 84-90, 2010.

Ghosh, S., DeCoffe, D., Brown, K., Rajendiran, E., Estaki, M., Dai, C., Yip, A., and Gibson, DL. Fish Oil Attenuates Omega-6 Polyunsaturated Fatty Acid-Induced Dysbiosis and Infectious Colitis but Impairs LPS Dephosphorylation Activity Causing Sepsis. *PLoS One*. 8(2): e55468, 2013.

Ghosh, S., Molcan, E., DeCoffe, D., Dai, C., and Gibson, DL. Diets Rich in n-6 PUFA Induce Intestinal Microbial Dysbiosis in Aged Mice. *Br J Nutr*. 110(3): 515-23, 2013.

Gregory, JC., Buffa, JA., Org, E, Wang, Z., Levison, BS., Zhu, W., Wagner, MA., Bennett, BJ., Li, L, DiDonato, JA., Lusis, AJ., and Hazen, SL. Transmission of Atherosclerosis Susceptibility with Gut Microbial Transplantation. *J Biol Chem*. 290(9): 5647-60, 2015.

Hawrelak, JA. The Causes of Intestinal Dysbiosis: A Review. *Alt Med Rev*. 9(2): 180-197, 2004.

Hasegawa, S., Goto, S., Tsuji, H., Okuno, T., Asahara, T., Nomoto, K., Shibata, A., Fujisawa, Y., Minato, T., Okamoto, A., Ohno, K., Hirayama, M. Intestinal Dysbiosis and Lowered Serum Lipopolysaccharide-Binding Protein in Parkinson's Disease. *PLoS One*. 10(11): e0142164, 2015.

Hildebrandt, MA., Hoffmann, C., Sherrill-Mix, SA., Keilbaugh, SA., Hamady, M., Chen, YY., Knight, R., Ahima, RS., Bushman, F., and Wu, GD. High-Fat Diet Determines the Composition of the Murine Gut Micro-biome Independently of Obesity. *Gastroenterology.* 137(5): 1716-24.e1-2, 2009.

Jakobsdottir, G., Xu, J., Molin, G., Ahrné, S., and Nyman, M. High-Fat Diet Reduces the Formation of Butyrate, but Increases Succinate, Inflammation, Liver Fat and Cholesterol in Rats, while Dietary Fibre Counteracts These Effects. *PLoS One.* 8(11): e80476, 2013.

Kaliannan, K., Wang, B., Li, XY., Kim, KJ., and Kang, JX. A Host-Microbiome Interaction Mediates the Opposing Effects of Omega-6 and Omega-3 Fatty Acids on Meta-bolic Endotoxemia. *Sci Rep.* 5: 11276, 2015.

Kankaanpää, PE., Salminen, SJ., Isolauri, E., and Lee, YK. The Influence of Polyunsaturated Fatty Acids on Probiotic Growth and Adhesion. *FEMS Microbiol Lett.* 194(2): 149-53, 2001.

Kimura, I., Inoue, D., Hirano, K., and Tsujimoto, G. The SCFA Receptor GPR43 and Energy Metabolism. *Front Endocrinol (Lausanne).* 5:85, 2014.

Koeth, RA., Wang, Z., Levison, BS., Buffa, JA., Org, E., Sheehy, BT., Britt, EB., Fu, X., Wu, Y., Li, L., Smith, JD., DiDonato, JA., Chen, J., Li, H., Wu, GD., Lewis, JD., Warrier, M., Brown, JM., Krauss, RM., Tang, WH., Bush-man, FD., Lusis, AJ., Hazen, SL. Intestinal Microbiota Metabolism of *L*-carnitine, a Nutrient in Red meat, Pro-motes Atherosclerosis. *Nat Med.* 19(5): 576-585, 2013.

Koren, O., Spor, A., Felin, J., Fåk, F., Stombaugh, J., Tremaroli, V., Behre, CJ., Knight, R., Fagerberg, B., Ley, RE., and Bäckhed, F. Human Oral, Gut, and Plaque Microbiota in Patients with Atherosclerosis. *Proc Natl Acad Sci*. 108 Suppl 1: 4592-8, 2011.

Litherland, GJ., Hajduch, E., Gould, GW., and Hundal, HS. Fructose Transport and Metabolism in Adipose Tissue of Zucker Rats: Diminished GLUT5 Activity During Obesity and Insulin Resistance. *Mol Cell Biochem*. 261(1-2): 23-33, 2004.

Mafra, D., Lobo, JC., Barros, AF., Koppe, L., Vaziri, ND., and Fouque, D. Role of Altered Intestinal Microbiota in Systemic Inflammation and Cardiovascular Disease in Chronic Kidney Disease Future. Microbiol. 9(3): 399-410, 2014.

Manco, M., Putignani, L., and Bottazzo, GF. Gut Microbiota, Lipopolysaccharides, and Innate Immunity in the Pathogenesis of Obesity and Cardiovascular Risk. *Endocrine Reviews* 31: 817-844, 2010.

McFarland, LV. Use of Probiotics to Correct Dysbiosis of Normal Microbiota Following Disease or Disruptive Events: A Systematic Review. *BMJ Open* 4: e005047, 2014.

Neves, AL., Coelho, J., Couto, L., Leite-Moreira, A., and Roncon-Albuquerque, R. Metabolic Endotoxemia: a Molecular Link Between Obesity and Cardiovascular Risk. *J Mo Endocrinol*. 51(2):R51-64, 2013.

Poutahidis, T., Cappelle, K., Levkovich, T., Lee, CW.,

Doulberis, M., Ge, Z., Fox, JG., Horwitz, BH., and Erd-
man, SE. Pathogenic Intestinal Bacteria Enhance Prostate Cancer Development via Systemic Activation of Immune Cells in Mice. *PLoS One*. 8(8):e73933, 2013.

Pluznick, JL., Protzko, RJ., Gevorgyan, H., Peterlin, Z.,
Sipos, A., Han, J., Brunet, I., Wan, LX., Rey, F., Wang, T.,
Firestein, SJ., Yanagisawa, M., Gordon, JI., Eichmann,
A., Peti-Peterdi, J., and Caplan, MJ. Olfactory Receptor
Responding to Gut Microbiota-Derived Signals Plays a
Role in Renin Secretion and Blood Pressure Regulation.
Proc Natl Acad Sci. 110(11): 4410-5, 2013.

Serino, M., Blasco-Baque, V., Nicolas, S., and Burcelin,
R. Far from the Eyes, Close to the Heart: Dysbiosis of
Gut Microbiota and Cardiovascular Consequences. *Curr
Cardiol Rep*. 16(11): 540, 2014.

Serrano, M., Moreno-Navarrete, JM., Puig, J., Moreno,
M., Guerra, E., Ortega, F., Xifra, G., Ricart, W., and Fer-
nández-Real, JM. Serum Lipopolysaccharide-binding
Protein as a Marker of Atherosclerosis. *Atherosclerosis*.
230(2):223-7, 2013.

Sobhani, I., Tap, J., Roudot-Thoraval, F., Roperch, JP.,
Letulle, S., Langella, P., Corthier, G., Tran Van Nhieu, J.,
and Furet, JP. Microbial Dysbiosis in Colorectal Cancer
(CRC) Patients. *PLoS One*. 6(1): e16393, 2011.

Tang, WH., Wang, Z., Levison, BS., Koeth, RA., Britt,
EB., Fu, X., Wu, Y., and Hazen, SL. Intestinal Microbial
Metabolism of Phosphatidylcholine and Cardiovascular
Risk. *N Engl J Med*. 368: 1575-84, 2013.

Tilg, H. and Moschen, AR. Microbiota and Diabetes: An

Evolving Relationship. *Gut*. 63(9): 1513-1521, 2014.

Tjonneland, A., Overvad, K., Bergmann, MM., Nagel, G., Linseisen, J., Hallmans, G., Palmqvist, R., Sjodin, H., Hagglund, G., Berglund, G., Lindgren, S., Grip, O., Palli, D., Day, NE., Khaw, KT., Bingham, S., Riboli, E., Kennedy, H., and Hart, A. Linoleic acid, a Dietary n-6 Polyunsaturated Fatty Acid, and the Etiology of Ulcerative Colitis: a Nested Case-Control Study within a European Prospective Cohort Study. *Gut* 58: 1606-1611, 2009.

Turnbaugh, PJ., Backhed, F., Fulton, L., and Gordon, JI. Marked Alterations in the Distal Gut Microbiome Linked to Diet Induced Obesity. *Cell Host Microbe*. 3(4): 213-223, 2008.

Westerterp, M., Berbée, JF., Pires, NM., van Mierlo, GJ., Kleemann, R., Romijn, JA., Havekes, LM., and Rensen, PC. Apolipoprotein C-I Is Crucially Involved in Lipopolysaccharide-Induced Atherosclerosis Development in Apolipoprotein E–Knockout Mice. *Circulation*. 116(19): 2173-81, 2007.

Zackular, JP., Baxter, NT., Iverson, KD., Sadler, WD., Petrosino, JF., Chen, GY., and Schloss, PD. The Gut Microbiome Modulates Colon Tumorigenesis. *MBio*. 4(6): e00692-13, 2013.

Zhang, YJ., Li, S., Gan, RY., Zhou. T., Xu, DP., and Li, HB. Impacts of Gut Bacteria on Human Health and Diseases. *Int J Mol Sci*. 16(4): 7493-519, 2015.

Chapter 10: Neurological Implications

Arimon, M., Takeda, S., Post, KL., Svirsky, S., Hyman, BT., and Berezovska, O. Oxidative Stress and Lipid Peroxidation are Upstream of Amyloid Pathology. *Neurobiol Dis*. pii: S0969-9961(15)00231-4, 2015.

Babu, GN., Kumar, A., Chandra, R., Puri, SK., Singh, RL., Kalita, J., and Misra, UK. Oxidant-Antioxidant Imbalance in the Erythrocytes of Sporadic Amyotrophic Lateral Sclerosis Patients Correlates with the Progression of Disease. *Neurochem Int*. 52(6): 1284-9, 2008.

Baillet, A., Chanteperdrix, V., Trocmé, C., Casez, P., Garrel, C., and Gérard Besson. The Role of Oxidative Stress in Amyotrophic Lateral Sclerosis and Parkinson's Disease. *Neurochem Res*. 35(10); 1530-1537, 2010.

Bredesen, DE. Reversal of Cognitive Decline: A Novel Therapeutic Program. *AGING*. 6(9), 2014.

Castellani, R., Hirai, K., Aliev, G., Drew, KL., Nunomura, A., Takeda, A., Cash, AD., Obrenovich, ME., Perry, G., and Smith, MA. Role of Mitochondrial Dysfunction in Alzheimer's disease. *J Neurosci Res*. 70(3): 357-60, 2002. Review

Chan, PH, and Fishman, RA. The Role of Arachidonic Acid in Vasogenic Brain Edema. *Fed Proc*. 43(2): 210-3, 1984.

Chan, PH., and Fishman, RA. Transient Formation of Superoxide Radicals in Polyunsaturated Fatty Acid-induced Brain Swelling. *J Neurochem*. 35(4): 1004-7, 1980.

Chan, PH., and Fishman, RA. Brain edema: Induction in Cortical Slices by Polyunsaturated Fatty Acids. *Science*.

201(4353): 358-60, 1978.

Fishman, RA., Caronna, J., Schmidley, JW., Prioleau, G., Lee, J. Induction of Brain Edema Following Intracerebral Injection of Arachidonic Acid. *Ann Neurol*. 13(6): 625-32, 1983.

Chan, PH., Fishman, RA., Lee, JL., and Quan, SC. Arachidonic Acid-Induced Swelling in Incubated Rat Brain Cortical Slices. Effect of Bovine Serum Albumin. *Neurochem Res*. 5(6): 629-40, 1980.

Chan, PH., Yurko, M., and Fishman, RA. Phospholipid Degradation and Cellular Edema Induced by Free Radicals in Brain Cortical Slices. *J Neurochem*. 38(2): 525-31, 1982.

Chan, PH., Fishman, RA., Schmidley, JW., and Chen, SF. Release of Polyunsaturated Fatty Acids from Phospholipids and Alteration of Brain Membrane Integrity by Oxygen-derived Free Radicals. *J Neurosci Res*. 12(4): 595-605, 1984.

Corrigan, FM., Horrobin, DF., Skinner, ER., Besson, JA., and Cooper, MB. Abnormal Content of n-6 and n-3 Long-chain Unsaturated Fatty Acids in the Phosphoglycerides and Cholesterol Esters of Parahippocampal Cortex from Alzheimer's Disease Patients and its Relationship to Acetyl CoA Content. *Int J Biochem Cell Biol*. 30(2): 197-207, 1998.

Dassati, S., Waldner, A., and Schweigreiter, R. Apolipoprotein D Takes Center Stage in the Stress Response of the Aging and Degenerative Brain. *Neurobiol Aging*.

35(7): 1632–1642, 2014.

Gamba, P., Testa, G., Gargiulo, S., Staurenghi, E., Poli, G., and Leonarduzzi, G. Oxidized Cholesterol as the Driving Force Behind the Development of Alzheimer's disease. *Aging Neurosci.* 7: 119, 2015.

Haider, L., Fischer, MT., Frischer, JM., Bauer, J., Höftberger, R., Botond, G., Esterbauer, H., Binder, CJ., Witztum, JL, and Lassmann, H. Oxidative Damage in Multiple Sclerosis Lesions. *Brain.* 134(Pt 7): 1914-24, 2011.

Hillered, L. and Chan, PH. Brain Mitochondrial Swelling Induced by Arachidonic Acid and Other Long Chain Free Fatty Acids. *J Neurosci Res.* 19(1):94-100, 1988.

Igarashi, M., Kim, H., Chang, L., Ma, K., and Rapoport, S. Dietary N-6 Polyunsaturated Fatty Acid Deprivation Increases Docosahexaenoic Acid Metabolism in Rat Bain. *J Neurochem.*120(6): 985–997, 2012.

Kim, H., Rao, J., Rapoport, S., and Igarashi. Dietary n-6 PUFA Deprivation Downregulates Arachidonate But Upregulates Docosahexaenoate Metabolizing Enzymes in Rat Brain. *Biochim Biophys Acta.* 1811(2): 111–117, 2011.

Lang-Lazdunski, L., Blondeau, N., Jarretou, G., Lazdunsk, M., and Heurteaux, C. Linolenic Acid Prevents Neuronal Cell Death and Paraplegia After Transient Spinal Cord Ischemia in Rats. *J Vasc Surg.* 38(3):564-75, 2003.

Lovell, M., Bradley, M., and Fister, S. 4-Hydroxyhexenal

(HHE) Impairs Glutamate Transport in Astrocyte Cultures. *Alzheimer's Dis*. 32(1): 139–146, 2012.

MacFabe, DF. Short-chain Fatty Acid Fermentation Products of the Gut Microbiome: Implications in Autism Spectrum Disorders. *Microb Ecol Health Dis*. 23: 19260, 2012.

McGrath, M.T., McGleenon, B.M., Brennan, S., McColl, D., McIlroy, S., and Passmore, A.P. Increased Oxidative Stress in Alzheimer's Disease as Assessed with 4-hydroxynonenal but not Malondialdhyde. *QJ Med*. 94: 485-490, 2001.

Melov, S., Adlard, PA., Morten, K., Johnson, F., Golden, TR., Hinerfeld, D., Schilling, B., Mavros, C., Masters, CL., Volitakis, I., Li, QX., Laughton, K., Hubbard, A., Cherny,. RA, Gibson, B., and Bush, AI. Mitochondrial Oxidative Stress Causes Hyperphosphorylation of Tau. *PLoS One*. 2(6): e536, 2007.

Michael-Titus, AT. Omega-3 Fatty Acids: Their Neuroprotective and Regenerative Potential in Traumatic Neurological Injury *Clin Lipidology*. 4(3): 343-353, 2009.

Miller, E., Morel, A., Saso, L., and Saluk, J. Isoprostanes and Neuroprostanes as Biomarkers of Oxidative Stress in Neurodegenerative Diseases. *Oxid Med Cell Longev*. 2014: 572491, 2014.

Newcombe J, Li H, and Cuzner ML. Low Density Lipoprotein Uptake by Macrophages in Multiple Sclerosis Plaques: Implications for Pathogenesis. *Neuropathol Appl Neurobiol*. 20(2): 152-62, 1994.

Perluigi, M., Fai Poon, H., Hensley, K., Pierce, WM., Klein, J.B., Calabrese, V., De Marco, C., and Butterfield, DA. Proteomic Analysis of 4-hydroxy-2-nonenal-modified Proteins in G93A-SOD1 Transgenic mice — A model of Familial Amyotrophic Lateral Sclerosis. *J Free Rad Biomed*, 38: 960– 968, 2005.

Picklo, MJ., Azenkeng, A., and Hoffmann, MR. *Trans*-4-oxo-2-nonenal Potently Alters Mitochondrial Function. *Free Radic Biol Med*. 50(2): 400-7, 2011.

Reddy, PH. Abnormal Tau, Mitochondrial Dysfunction, Impaired Axonal Transport of Mitochondria, and Synaptic Deprivation in Alzheimer's Disease. *Brain Res*. 1415: 136-48, 2011.

Ryu, JK., Cho, T., Choi, HB., Jantaratnotai, N., and McLarnon, JG. Pharmacological Antagonism of Interleukin-8 Receptor CXCR2 Inhibits Inflammatory Reactivity and is Neuroprotective in an Animal Model of Alzheimer's Disease. *J Neuroinflammation*. 12: 144, 2015.

Sultana, R, Perluigi, M., and Butterfield, D.A. Lipid Peroxidation Triggers Neurodegeneration: A Redox Proteomics View into the Alzheimer Disease Brain. *Free Radic Biol Med*. 62: 157–169, 2013.

Shoeb, M., Ansari, N., Srivastava, S., and Ramana, K. 4-hydroxynonenal in the Pathogenesis and Progression of Human Diseases. Curr Med Chem. 21(2): 230–237, 2014.

Whelan, J. (n-6) and (n-3) Polyunsaturated Fatty Acids and the Aging Brain: Food for Thought. *J Nutr*. 138: 2521–2522, 2008.

Yang, DY., Pan, HC., Yen, YJ., Wang, CC., Chuang, YH., Chen, SY., Lin, SY., Liao, SL., Raung, SL., Wu, CW., Chou, MC., Chiang, AN., and Chen, CJ. Detrimental Effects of Post-treatment with Fatty Acids on Brain Injury in Ischemic Rats. *Neurotoxicology*. 28(6): 1220-9. Epub 2007.

Yao, J., Irwin, RW., Zhao, L., Nilsen, J., Hamilton, RT., and Brinton, RD. Mitochondrial Bioenergetic Deficit Precedes Alzheimer's Pathology in Female Mouse Model of Alzheimer's Disease. *Proc Natl Acad Sci* 106(34):14670-5, 2009.

Yehuda, S. Omega–6/Omega–3 Ratio and Brain-Related Functions World *Rev Nutr Diet*. 92: 37–56, 2003.

Zhao, W., Wang J., Varghese, M., Hoi, L., Mazzola, P., Katsel, P., Gibson, G., Levine, S. Dubner, L., and Pasinette, G. Impaired Mitochondrial Energy Metabolism as a Novel Risk Factor for Selective Onset and Progression of Dementia in Oldest-old Subjects. *Neuropsychiatr Dis Treat*. 11: 565-74, 2015.

Chapter 11: Lipofuscin and Aging

Ames, BN., Shigenaga, MK., and Hagen, TM. Mitochondrial Decay in Aging. Biochim Biophys Acta. 1271(1):165-70, 1995.

Berger, HM., Den, Ouden, AL., and Calame, JJ. Pathogenesis of liver damage during parenteral nutrition: Is lipofuscin a clue? Arch Dis Child. 60(8):774-6, 1985.

Blaauboer, AJ., Novak, L. and Hooghwinkel, GJ. Neuronal Pigmented Autophagic Vacuoles: Lipofuscin, Neuromelanin, and Ceroid as Macroautophagic Responses During Aging and Disease. J Neurochem. 106(1):24-36, 2008.

Bronnikov GE, Kulagina TP, Aripovsky AV. Dietary Supplementation of Old Rats with Hydrogenated Peanut Oil Restores Activities of Mitochondrial Respiratory Complexes in Skeletal Muscles. Biochemistry (Mosc). 75(12):1491-7, 2010.

Brunk, UT. and Terman, A. Lipofuscin: Mechanisms of Age-related Accumulation and Influence on Cell Function. Free Radic Biol Med. 33(5):611-9, 2002.

Castro, Mdel R., Suarez, E., Kraiselburd, E., Isidro, A., Paz, J., Ferder, L., and Ayala-Torres, S. Aging Increases Mitochondrial DNA Damage and Oxidative Stress in Liver of Rhesus Monkeys. Exp Gerontol. 47(1):29-37, 2012.

Church, MW., Jen, KL., Anumba, JI., Jackson, DA., Adams, BR., and Hotra, JW. Excess Omega-3 Fatty Acid Consumption by Mothers During Pregnancy and Lactation Caused Shorter Life Span and Abnormal ABRs in Old Adult Offspring. Neurotoxicol Teratol. 32(2):171-81. Epub 2009 Oct 7.

Cole, GM., Ma, QL., and Frautschy, SA. Dietary Fatty Acids and the Aging Brain. Nutr Rev. 68 Suppl 2: S102-11, 2010.

Durand,. G, and Desnoyers, F. Polyunsaturated Fatty Acids and Aging. Lipofuscins : Structure, Origin and

Development. Ann Nutr Aliment. 34(2):317-32, 1980.

Giaccone, G., Orsi, L., Cupidi, C., and Tagliavini, F. Lipofuscin Hypothesis of Alzheimer's Disease. Dement Geriatr Cogn Dis Extra. 1(1):292-6, 2011.

Grigorov, IuG., Kozlovskaia, SG., Semes'ko, TM., and Asadov, ShA. Characteristics of Actual Nutrition of the Long-lived Population of Azerbaijan. Vopr Pitan. (2):36-40, 1991.

Guerra, A., Demmelmair, H., Toschke, AM, and Koletzko, B. Three-year Tracking of Fatty Acid Composition of Plasma Phospholipids in Healthy Children. Ann Nutr Metab. 51(5):433-8. Epub 2007.

Hochschild R. Effect of Dimethylaminoethyl p-chlorophenoxyacetate on the Life Span of Male Swiss Webster Albino Mice. Exp Gerontol. 8(4):177-83, 1973.

Harman, D. Lipofuscin and Ceroid Formation: The Cellular Recycling System. Adv Exp Med Biol. 266:3-15, 1989.

Hulbert AJ. Explaining Longevity of Different Animals: Is Membrane Fatty Acid Composition the Missing Link? Age. 30:89–97, 2008.

Hulbert AJ., Faulks, SC., and Buffenstein, R. Oxidation-resistant Membrane Phospholipids Can Explain Longevity Differences Among the Longest-living Rodents and Similarly-sized Mice. J Gerontol A Biol Sci Med Sci. 61(10):1009-18, 2006.

Hulbert, AJ., Pamplona, R., Buffenstein, R, and

Buttemer. WA. Life and Death: Metabolic Rate, Membrane Composition, and Life Span of Animals. Physiol Rev. 87(4):1175-213, 2007.

Kennedy, CJ., Rakoczy, PE., and Constable, IJ. Lipofuscin of the Retinal Pigment Epithelium: A Review. Eye (Lond). 9 (Pt 6):763-71, 1996.

Koobs, DH., Schultz, RL., and Jutzy, RV. The Origin of Lipofuscin and Possible Consequences to the Myocardium. Arch Pathol Lab Med. 1978 Feb;102(2):66-8.

Kunkel, HO., and Williams, JN. The Effects of Fat Deficiency Upon Enzyme Activity in the Rat. J Biol Chem. 1951 Apr;189(2):755-61.

Laganiere, S. and Yu, BP. Anti-lipoperoxidation Action of Food Restriction. Biochem Biophys Res Commun. 145(3):1185-91, 1987.

Laganiere S. and Yu BP. Modulation of Membrane Phospholipid Fatty Acid Composition by Age and Food Restriction. Gerontology. 39(1):7-18, 1993.

Lee, HJ., Mayette, J., Rapoport, SI., and Bazinet, RP. Selective Remodeling of Cardiolipin Fatty Acids in the Aged Rat Heart. Lipids Health Dis. 23;5:2, 2006.

Lee, J., Yu, BP., and Herlihy, JT. Modulation of Cardiac Mitochondrial Membrane Fluidity by Age and Calorie Intake. Free Radic Biol Med. 1999 Feb;26(3-4):260-5.

Mann, DM. and Yates, PO. Accumulation of Lipoprotein Pigments in Nerve Cells of British and Sri Lankan nationals. Mech Ageing Dev. 18(2):151-8, 1982.

Mitchell, TW., Buffenstein, R., and Hulbert, AJ. Membrane Phospholipid Composition May Contribute to Exceptional Longevity of the Naked Mole-rat (Heterocephalus glaber): A Comparative Study Using Shotgun Lipidomics. Exp Gerontol. 42(11):1053-62, 2007.

Nowak, JZ. Oxidative Stress, Polyunsaturated Fatty Acids Derived Oxidation Products and Bisretinoids as Potential Inducers of CNS diseases: Focus on Age-related Macular Degeneration. Pharmacological Reports. 65, 288.304, 2013.

Nourooz-Zadeh J, Pereira P. Age-related Accumulation of Free Polyunsaturated Fatty Acids in Human Retina. Ophthalmic Res. 31(4):273-9, 1999.

Paradies G, Ruggiero FM, Petrosillo G, Quagliariello E. Age-dependent Decline in the Cytochrome C Oxidase Activity in Rat Heart Mitochondria: Role of Cardiolipin. FEBS Lett. 406(1-2):136-8, 1997.

Riga, S. and Riga, D. Effects of Centrophenoxine on the Lipofuscin Pigments in the Nervous System of Old Rats. Brain Res. 72(2):265-75, 1974.

Schäfer, L., Overvad, K., Thorling, EB., and Velander, G. Adipose Tissue Levels of Fatty Acids and Tocopherol in Young and Old Women. Ann Nutr Metab. 33(6):315-22, 1989.

Skoumalová, A., Mádlová, P., and Topinková, E. End Products of Lipid Peroxidation in Erythrocyte Membranes in Alzheimer's Disease. Cell Biochem Funct. 30(3):205-10, 2012.

Solfrizzi, V., D'Introno, A., Colacicco, AM., Capurso, C., Palasciano, R., Capurso, S., Torres, F., Capurso, A., and Panza, F. Unsaturated Fatty Acids Intake and All-causes Mortality: A 8.5-year Follow-up of the Italian Longitudinal Study on Aging. Exp Gerontol. 40(4):335-43, 2005.

Sulzer, D., Mosharov, E., Talloczy, Z., Zucca, FA., Simon, JD., and Zecca, L. Neuronal Pigmented Autophagic Vacuoles: Lipofuscin, Neuromelanin, and Ceroid as Macroautophagic Responses During Aging and Disease. J Neurochem. 106(1):24-36, 2008.

Tamburini, I., Quartacci, MF., Izzo, R., and Bergamini, E. Effects of Dietary Restriction on Age-related Changes in the Phospholipid Fatty Acid Composition of Various Rat Tissues. Aging Clin Exp Res. 2004 Dec;16(6):425-31.

Terman, A. and Brunk, UT. The Aging Myocardium: Roles of Mitochondrial Damage and Lysosomal Degradation. Heart Lung Circ. 14(2):107-14, 2005.

Terman, A., Kurz, T., Navratil, M., Arriaga, EA., and Brunk, UT. Mitochondrial Turnover and Aging of Long-Lived Postmitotic Cells: The Mitochondrial–Lysosomal Axis Theory of Aging. Antioxidants & Redox Signaling. Volume 12, Number 4, 2010.

Valencak, TG. and Azzu, V. Making Heads or Tails of Mitochondrial Membranes in Longevity and Aging: A Role for Comparative Studies. Longevity & Health span 3:3, 2014.